D0932943

# YogaMass

Embodying Christ Consciousness

## Gena Davis

Foreword by J. Pittman McGehee, D.D.

**BALBOA.**
PRESS

A DIVISION OF HAY HOUSE

Scripture quotations marked NRSV are taken from the New Revised Standard Version of the Bible, Copyright © 1989, by the Division of Christian Education of the National Council of the Churches of Christ in the United States of America. Used by permission. All rights reserved. Website: http://www.nrsv.net

Balboa Press books may be ordered through booksellers or by contacting:

Balboa Press
A Division of Hay House
1663 Liberty Drive
Bloomington, IN 47403
www.balboapress.com
1 (877) 407-4847

Because of the dynamic nature of the Internet, any web addresses or links contained in this book may have changed since publication and may no longer be valid. The views expressed in this work are solely those of the author and do not necessarily reflect the views of the publisher, and the publisher hereby disclaims any responsibility for them.

The author of this book does not dispense medical advice or prescribe the use of any technique as a form of treatment for physical, emotional, or medical problems without the advice of a physician, either directly or indirectly. The intent of the author is only to offer information of a general nature to help you in your quest for emotional and spiritual well-being. In the event you use any of the information in this book for yourself, which is your constitutional right, the author and the publisher assume no responsibility for your actions.

Printed in the USA

ISBN: 978-1-5043-7775-1 (sc)
ISBN: 978-1-5043-7777-5 (hc)
ISBN: 978-1-5043-7776-8 (e)

Library of Congress Control Number: 2017904836

Balboa Press rev. date: 05/26/2017

# Contents

# Acknowledgements

With heartfelt gratitude and love, I wish to thank my husband, Gary Davis, for your tireless patience, love and support. Thank you for always being here with me and for me. Your steadfast love has made this book and my life work possible.

A special thank you to my father, Richard Lassmann, for teaching me to believe in myself and to persevere in what you know is right and true; and to my mother, Margie Lassmann, for showing me alternative modalities of health and encouraging me to follow my heart always.

Of particular importance, I am grateful for the loving community of Grace Episcopal Church, Houston, who gave me love, space, and time to follow my heart. I wish to thank The Reverend Dr. John K. Graham for your encouragement to write this book, and for your partnership in YogaMass® as a heart offering and a bridge for spiritual, emotional, and physical healing. I wish to thank The Very Reverend J. Pittman McGehee, D.D., for your encouragement and wise counsel, and your insights into Jungian psychology and the theology of becoming. I would also like to thank Julie Clayton for your wonderful and gentle support, editing, and feedback. I wish to thank The Reverend Dr. Richard Kleiman for your encouragement, feedback, and laughter. I wish to thank my many yoga teachers who have led me on the journey of my lifetime into the depths of spiritual awakening in my body to a higher consciousness, especially Don and Amba Stapleton, Robert Boustany, and Sharon Kapp. I wish to thank Swami Kesava Bharati Das Goswami for sharing your truth and devotional love with me, and Dr. Hansa Medley of the International Society for Krishna Consciousness (ISKCON) for your continued enthusiasm and encouragement. I especially wish to thank The Right Reverend C. Andrew Doyle, IX Bishop of the Episcopal Diocese of Texas, for your open heart and willingness to allow me to be creative in spiritual leadership and sharing the sacramental life. I also wish to thank The Reverend Dr. Stephen Kinney of the Front Porch in Austin, Texas, for sharing your liturgy that brings our worship into a close and personal relationship with the divine.

I am grateful to all of you who bring your talents and service so that we can offer YogaMass, especially the Institute for Spirituality and Health at the Texas Medical Center team: Stuart Nelson for your encouragement and soulful sitar playing during YogaMass; Cyrus Wirls for your boundless enthusiasm and energetic drumming; and Lex Gillan for your guidance and wisdom in integrating yoga and meditation into the worship experience. I am particularly grateful to the Grace Episcopal Church musicians and singers (especially Diane Davis Andrew for your leadership) for your input on the liturgy, flow, and musical components of the worship experience, and to CJ Rubenak, for offering your gifts of yoga teacher and wisdom to the YogaMass experience. I wish to thank everyone at Grace Episcopal Church in Houston who helps to offer YogaMass worship so we can connect to God in this spiritually embodied way.

To the YogaMass participants, thank you for allowing me the opportunity to share the teachings of yoga and Christ with you. And to my yoga students who allow me to teach you, you bless me.

Deep bow to you all.

# Foreword

My colleague, Gena Davis, and I have for some time been in dialogue about wholeness. There are four aspects to the "whole" human being; we humans are Bio-Psycho-Social-Spiritual beings. This book seeks to explicate and integrate these four natures of human wholeness when on the path of deepening one's spiritual life.

My definition of spirituality is the deep human longing to transfer the Transcendent into the Immanent through experience and reflection upon it. The Reverend Ms. Davis uses spiritual practices from different traditions to develop the four natures of human wholeness. The novel idea that one could integrate yogic practices with the Christian Sacrament of Eucharist as a spiritual ritual of wholeness called YogaMass® is soul food for anyone seeking to experience the Presence of the Transcendent. YogaMass engages body, soul, and community, providing a container for experiencing the kingdom within, and for integrating the four natures of the whole person. The Buddhist tradition holds that "enlightenment is always accidental, but spiritual practice makes one accident prone!"

This book is a significant contribution to one of the most important conversations of the 21st Century. That being, "What are the resources for experiencing The Source of the Mystery?" This book is such a resource!

–The Very Reverend J. Pittman McGehee, D.D.

Author of *Extraordinary in the Ordinary; The Invisible Church: Finding Spirituality Where You Are (Psychology, Religion, and Spirituality); Paradox of Love; Words Made Flesh: Selected Sermons by The Very Reverend J. Pittman McGehee D.D.; Growing Down;* and *Raising Lazarus: The Science of Healing the Soul*

# Preface

*If you love God and you love yoga, this book is for you. Welcome. You don't have to practice yoga in secret, wondering if you are being unfaithful to your religious beliefs or tradition, even if you are a Christian. A Christian myself, and an ordained Episcopal priest, I have also studied and practiced yoga, and discovered that its ancient truths are compatible with Christian beliefs. You see, yoga itself is not a religion or a belief system, although inherent in its teachings is a path to the depths of a spiritual life in the human experience.*

*Yoga is an ancient philosophy, developed over 5,000 years ago. It was explored and explained through the lens of both the Hindu and the Buddhist traditions because of its origination in India, although it predates both of these religions. Many people mistakenly believe that yoga is part of the Hindu religion, or the Buddhist philosophy. Yoga is actually the science of human experience, explained and illumined initially by Hinduism, and later Buddhism, as those were the religions of the peoples in the country where the science of yoga originated. As a science, yoga facilitates connection to the highest truth and awakens greater awareness and connection to self and life.*

*As we journey together, I will lead you through my personal discovery of how yoga provides a path for knowing oneself—and for the seeker of wisdom and truth, yoga also offers a spiritual path for seeking the divine that Christians and people of many faiths can embrace. A spiritual path flows naturally out of the human experience, because we humans are spiritual beings. Yoga does not change or negate one's religious beliefs; instead, the science and practice of yoga can be a bridge between the understanding of self and a path to the divine, which Jesus refers to as the kingdom of heaven. As Jesus said, come and see.*

# Introduction

## This is my body

*This is my body.* Upon hearing these words, while flowing through a series of standing yoga postures, it all became crystal clear. It was one of those *aha* moments in life. It felt as if the heavens had opened up and downloaded clarity into my whole being. *This is my body.*

These were the words spoken by Jesus on the last night of his life, with his friends at dinner, when he instituted a new way of being in community, in relationship, with his presence. *"This is my body, given for you"* (Luke 22:19).

These are the words spoken in the Eucharistic prayer by the priest, remembering Jesus and following his commandment to "do this as often as you can, in remembrance of me." *This is my body.*

These are the words spoken by my yoga teacher, Amba Stapleton, her voice ringing clear as she leads our group of 40 in teacher training and guides us through vigorous and energizing movements. *"This is my body."*

## Integration

On the first night of yoga teacher training, each participant was asked to write down a word or phrase next to our photo that described our intention for the next 28 days. My word was *integration*. I knew that in the days ahead of me, training in the warm, humid jungle of Costa Rica would be demanding physically and psychologically, but even beyond my obvious limitations, I knew deep down that the most challenging component would be spiritual.

You see, I am a Christian, and I am an ordained Episcopal priest, and yet surprisingly yoga had spoken to me as deeply as the sacraments I have been ordained to administer on behalf of the Christian church for the people of God. So my word was *integration*. I needed, on the soul level, to find a way to integrate the gifts of the scientific and spiritual practice and truths of yoga into my spiritual life as a practicing and faithful Christian. It felt risky, scary, adventurous, and one of the most exciting journeys I had ever embarked on! And it felt so right, so necessary, so inescapable for my own soul to pursue this path as my path to authenticity.

## My Body, Your Body

This is my body. Each and every one of us can say this unequivocally—some more hesitantly and some more joyfully than others. Our bodies are unique and there is no other exactly like ours on the entire planet.

For many women, our bodies are a constant reminder of how we are "never good enough," according to much of modern media's messaging. We think we must look like the women in the glamour magazines: tall, thin, perfect hair, skin, and teeth made even more perfect with photo manipulations. As a teenager, and like most teenagers today, I believed I needed to be more like those images and less like who I actually was. I did love to wear those platform shoes of the 70s! Over time, however, I came to love the shoes that made my feet feel good rather than those that supposedly made me look taller, thinner, and sexier.

For men, body image is important too, although they receive different body messages than women. Men constantly live under the pressure of being perceived as weak,[1] which is culturally judged as "less than" masculine. Physical strength, stature, and body image are important factors in how a man views himself and his place in the world.

Both men and women need affirmation that our bodies are desirable. Not just attractive to potential partners, but desirable in terms of being healthy, vital, and strong, so that we feel good about ourselves. These days we have access to a plethora of information reminding us that exercise and a healthy lifestyle makes a significant difference in the shape, strength, and well-being of our bodies, and that we each need to take care of our physical being.

Whether the emphasis on our physicality is superficial or health-driven, there is an underlying truth that seems to have been lost in our culture: *our bodies are beautiful.* No matter what size or shape, our bodies are handmade by God, with the genetics of our biological parents and ancestors. Our features may not be model-perfect, but they are nonetheless perfect. The gift of being alive begins with knowing your body and being comfortable in your body, regardless of your body's particular shape, size, color of skin, and even imperfections. It took me many years to discover this perspective, and as my spiritual life blossomed, it gradually became my truth.

Whether one thinks that we are spiritual beings having a human experience, or physical beings having a spiritual experience, we cannot deny that we are in these bodies. Our bodies are the vehicles for expression in this life. One of my yoga teachers in Houston, Robert Boustany, yoga master and developer of the Pralaya Yoga System, taught me a simple and yet profound truth: *Your body will teach you everything.* This sounds somewhat mysterious, but actually is very profound. Over the years I have come to realize the ways in which "my body" has been one of my greatest spiritual teachers. The gift of being alive in this body is to experience life through it—to embody it completely and fully. And if I listen closely to what my body—not just my mind—is telling me, I hear *my* truth.

As we journey together in this exploration of knowing our whole selves, including our bodies, it is helpful to distinguish the uses of mind, soul, and spirit. I am grateful for the work of Cyprian Consiglio, American Camaldolese Benedictine monk, musician, and spiritual teacher, whom I first met at a World Community for Christian Meditation seminar. He gave me great insight and inspiration for integrating these words and ideas.

I use the word soul in the context of consciousness and intuition as Consiglio defines it:

> "Our soul is the inner realm, matter coming into consciousness, and then coming into self-consciousness and learning to harness the powers of the mind."[2]

For Consiglio, the mind is distinguishable from soul in this informative way:

> "Perhaps the rational mind is at the center, but it is surrounded by all the strata of the soul, the *psyche*—the subconscious, higher states of consciousness, the collective unconscious, and psychic powers and phenomena of all sorts."[3]

I will use the terms heart, body, mind, soul and spirit throughout this book, with the understanding that the mind is the rational mind, and the soul is a broader aspect of ourselves, including emotions, intuition, and personality. The term *heart* is the seat of the soul, and I will be using *heart* to refer to the organ of cosmic intuition and perception. I will also use Consiglio's understanding of the human spirit as the eternal self, the inner person, the spirit, the spark of divinity within the soul, having the potential to open to the Spirit of God—and to the ultimate union with God and the Holy Spirit. These distinctions within ourselves are important in understanding the subtleties of addressing the whole person; even more important is understanding the inseparability of our body from the other aspects of our human being-ness.

Through yoga and other eastern practices such as Tai Chi and Qigong, Christians are beginning to rediscover the experience of God through our bodies and our senses. Yoga has brought a depth to the self-exploration of my body, as well as my heart and my mind. As a physical practice, yoga postures raise energy, strengthen and stretch muscles, align the skeletal structure, open connective tissue, increase circulation, bring blood supply to the organs, and release repressed emotions. As a spiritual practice, yoga raises consciousness with every breath, calms the mind, and increases awareness of divine presence. Yoga is a science that provides a path for spiritual transformation and achieving higher levels of consciousness of the ultimate reality of divine presence. Physical Yoga was primarily designed to facilitate the true practice of Yoga, which was the understanding and complete mastery of the mind so that spiritual transformation would be possible.

The gradual understanding of the inseparability of my whole self—body, mind, soul, and spirit—eventually led me to the blending of eastern energetic practices into my western faith tradition, and the integration gave rise to a new expression of spiritual ritual and celebration called "YogaMass®."

The purpose of this book is to introduce how, by bridging yogic principles and practices into a practice of embodied Christian spirituality, one can discover the kingdom of God within and open the whole self to the experience of spiritual awakening and transformation into Christ Consciousness.

Since we are largely disconnected from our bodies—especially in a spiritual sense—the practice of yoga is a way to reconnect to what the body can teach us, and it provides a vital understanding and methodology for integrating the body, mind, soul, and spirit for a holistic approach to life that includes offering our bodies as vehicles for spiritual service. Our bodies are vehicles to experience God in them, as them, and through them, and integrating our bodies into the worship experience and the sacredness of daily life reconnects us to the presence of God as indwelling Spirit.

A key component of Christian love is to serve. Our bodies help us to serve with love. Our bodies are vessels for God's Spirit to dwell. Our bodies are the vehicles for our souls to take action— for devotion and service. Awareness of our bodies as part of our very created-ness leads to accepting our bodies as having worth, of being beautiful, and the opportunity for offering them in a spiritual sense.

To fully appreciate the body is to understand that our bodies are our sacred temples for life, love, and service, as St. Paul understood: "Do you not know that your body is a temple of the Holy Spirit within you, which you have from God, and that you are not your own?" (1 Corinthians 6:19). Therefore, to honor our bodies is a sacred thing, and to do so brings fullness and wholeness to the Christian life. A temple is a "building devoted to the worship of God," or alternatively, a "house of prayer." How might our faith be more whole or enhanced when the body becomes a holy house of prayer?

## Finding Joy in the Body

The spiritual path evolves over a lifetime. Our bodies offer different experiences, depending on our age along with our physical, emotional, and spiritual wellness. Before discovering yoga, I have always loved to move my body, and I had a keen sense that when I am moving, I feel good, I feel alive. When I sit still too long I become lethargic, and my body becomes sore. I feel restored, rejuvenated, balanced when I allow my body to move.

As a child, I ran, rode my bike like the wind, climbed trees. I ran barefoot as often as I could. As a teenager, I was a twirler with the marching band, practicing skills and choreographed routines for up to four hours a day after school, until it got too dark to see. I ran track in high school, preferring the longer and more paced distances, enjoying getting into the rhythm of breath and movement. I found peace on the trails. In retrospect, I realize that all this movement was "soul movement."

I call it soul movement because even as a youth, I could feel a deep, wordless joy when I moved my body. As a teenager and young adult, I loved to go to clubs and rock concerts and dance, dance, dance. I danced as often as possible. Dancing made me feel free. I lost myself in the rhythm of the beat, and I was able to let go of thoughts that bound me and kept me small. The dancing moved me into a liminal space of freedom and possibilities. I didn't need a dance partner, and often I just danced alone or with friends. Much later in life I discovered the wonderful way that Asian Indians dance—in a circle, everyone together, often with some lucky person in the middle of the circle. I love this form of dancing—it isn't the Western style where everyone needs a partner. It is freeform; anyone can join in, and all are welcome. All are invited to join in the movement, the joy, and the ecstasy. No judgment, simply joy.

I began practicing yoga while in high school, back in the late 1970s, with a teacher named Lilias, who offered a Hatha Yoga class on the Public Broadcasting Service television channel (PBS). I felt alive when I practiced the movements along with her. Even more, I felt peace and serenity. But my interest fell away with my studies and pursuit of my career. In the dark recesses of my memory, I always remembered the gift of that short and sweet practice—it hauntingly and lovingly stayed with me.

Fast-forward 25 years. After an intense and rewarding career in human resources and information systems, a broken heart, the joys of motherhood, my second marriage, and new healthy relationships, I landed back in Austin to attend the Episcopal Seminary of the Southwest, on the road to the ordination to the priesthood. It seemed a whirlwind of Holy Spirit movement (again, "soul movement"), leading the way for me and opening doors I never dreamed I would walk through.

## Finding Spirituality in the Body

While attending seminary in Austin, Texas in my mid-forties, my spiritual nourishment came with the balance of experiencing God through daily worship and daily meditation. I led a contemplative prayer group my last two years of seminary to share the gift of the silence of the heart with others. To my happy surprise, I rediscovered yoga and began to learn Tai Chi. At a nearby yoga studio on Guadalupe Street near the University of Texas campus, I entered into a deep spiritual practice which integrated sacred texts, physical movement, music, incense, and compassion in community under the leadership of two spirit-filled human beings. This was a surprising encounter, as I was already in a spirit-filled community in training to lead Christian communities of faith. But my mat drew me in and down, into my body and into my soul, and it was on my mat that I found a deep sense of nurturing, peace, and grounding, which enabled me to go back into the academic world with a deeper connection to the process of preparation for the priesthood, and a deeper connection with myself and with God.

There was just one problem: the practice of yoga created an internal conflict within me. Inner challenges, struggles, and dilemmas have never been new to me, but this was different. My challenge was that the yoga being taught used Buddhist and Hindu teachings to enhance the practice and add a spiritual dimension. I was plagued with a vague and nagging feeling that I was somehow being unfaithful to my Christian roots.

Then to my surprise, one of the teachers played Christian chants during long, slow holds of yoga poses, and that helped me feel safe and grounded. She played a beautiful rendition of the song *Ave Maria* that brought tears flowing down my face. I didn't talk about my yoga practice at seminary because I felt as though I would be judged as "wrong" and disloyal to my faith tradition. Yet it felt so right to move my body, and flow in the yoga poses. Even though I had questions about yoga being in conflict with Christian beliefs, the yoga practice continued to draw me in. When I would discover a parallel of the ethics and spiritual truths between yogic practices and Christianity, I felt joy and relief. But still my yoga practice gnawed at me, as if I were somehow "breaking the rules."

I was most concerned with being faithful, honest and true to my religion and the church that was raising me to serve in community. But inside my body and soul, I knew that what was happening to me on my mat was life changing and good. I could not deny its value and worth to me—as a spiritual being having a human experience.

In my second year of seminary, a redemptive moment occurred. A classmate organized a meeting with a small group of women seminarian students and our female mentor and New Testament professor, who is now the Dean of the Seminary of the Southwest, The Very Reverend Cynthia Briggs Kittredge. After breaking bread together, we went into the chapel that was filled with afternoon sunlight, and we intentionally acknowledged our souls and our bodies in the space. Each of us spoke the words that Jesus spoke on the night before he died, *"This is my body,"* each with our own feminine voice. Dean Kittredge, our teacher and guide, gave us courage to simply trust, with fearless hearts, our call to the ordained priesthood, as women. I asked her about her Sunday morning preparations before presiding at the Lord's Table, and her words, unknowingly, affirmed my heart in a profound way. "Pray, do yoga, open," she said. With these few, simple words, I was set free.

After settling into my new position in a church, I followed my heart and enrolled in yoga teacher training in Houston, but couldn't complete it due to my demanding ministry schedule. My teacher knew that I was an Episcopal priest and that I felt anxious and yet excited about being in a teacher-training course. It took three more years for me to finally dive in and complete my first 200 hours of yoga teacher training. By then, I knew deep in my heart that my yoga practice was consistent with my Christian contemplative prayer practice. True, certain beliefs were different when religious stories and myths were shared, but the goal of *union with God* is the same for most faith traditions. So I wholeheartedly committed to integrating yoga into my personal spiritual practice, knowing that God was calling me to go deeper. Earlier in the same year, a creative friend, formerly an Episcopal priest, Lyndon Harris, nudged me with enthusiasm and a great big smile when he learned I was enrolled for yoga teacher training. He said so clearly and decisively, "You can create a new service called 'YogaMass'. It will integrate yoga into the Christian ritual of Holy Communion." At that moment of great clarity, the heavens opened up and I felt as if God had spoken directly to me through Lyndon. "Yes!"

## Life with God in the Body

As I was creating YogaMass, a Eucharist service integrating yoga, meditation and breath work, it felt as though I was being propelled forward with momentum and an invisible force, which I had no doubt was the Holy Spirit at work. Doors opened, seemingly effortlessly. A friend and my Bishop's Warden at Grace Episcopal Church, Philip Montgomery, set up a planning lunch with an Episcopal Priest and medical doctor, The Reverend Dr. John K. Graham, the President and CEO of the Institute for Spirituality and Health at the Texas Medical Center in Houston.

When we told him about the creation of YogaMass, John's face lit up with joy and excitement. He immediately offered to partner with us and I can truthfully say, the rest is history. John and his staff warmly embraced the essence of this new form of worship as an offering of both spirituality and health to a wider community, with Grace Episcopal Church as our home base.

At the first meeting the following Monday, two staff members of the Institute volunteered wholeheartedly to be the musicians for the service: Cyrus Wirls on djembe drums and Stuart Nelson on sitar. Vocalists at Grace volunteered to lead Taizé-style singing during Holy Communion, under the direction of Christian folk singer/songwriter Diane Davis Andrew. The collaboration between the Institute for Spirituality and Health (ISH) and Grace Episcopal Church, Houston, came from a mutual desire to manifest Christ Consciousness in the world, through a marriage of sacred meal and mat, east and west, movement and stillness, body and breath.

As we began to offer YogaMass, excitement spread. The Holy Spirit indeed was up to something, and the best I could do was flow and try to relax and have fun with the new thing God was doing. When I spoke about YogaMass, people were inspired. People who attended YogaMass were inspired. They encouraged my courageousness and pioneering spirit (some even calling it "heroic," likening the birthing process to my own heroine's journey). I was told that when I talked about YogaMass, my face lit up and I exuded joy—which is one of the greatest gifts of the Holy Spirit.

The spirituality of YogaMass is embodied, conscious, and fully human. My vision is to bring everyone to know the love and light of Christ, and to become that light through an integral approach on the mat of yoga, meditation, breath work, and Holy Communion. Holy Communion brings us to the promise of Jesus of the "kingdom of God within," and the integral approach of practicing Christian spirituality inclusive of yoga offers a path to awakening to this divine reality. In seeking God, we discover through yogic practices the inner spark of divinity and creative energy within ourselves, opening up to the higher consciousness that Jesus embodied in his life.

An integral approach to discovering the "kingdom of God within" and awakening to Christ Consciousness, as I am offering it, consists of an embodied human experience and focuses on spiritual communion with Christ through sacred ritual and yogic practices. I use the term "integral" to describe the approach of bridging yogic practices into Christian spirituality, basing it on a key insight from Ken Wilber, American philosopher and writer, and creator of his own Integral Theory, who understands "integral" to mean a comprehensive and inclusive synthesis of all human knowledge and experience.

Through the exploration of an integral approach that bridges yogic practices into the Christian life, I hope to show how yoga's philosophy, understanding, and practices can deepen the spirituality of a Christian, on and off the mat. As Christians, we can discover an awakening or realization of divine presence in many ways—one of which is yoga. Throughout this book, as I use the term "awakening," I am defining "awakening" as a realization and intimate touching of the divine.

I will share with you the sacred journey of developing YogaMass, which is founded on an integral approach to spirituality and faith, and the theological foundation for its birth emerging from my own journey with yoga as a Christian and as a priest ordained in The Episcopal Church. Each chapter of this book reflects the various personal and spiritual elements that sustain an integral approach that allows us to bring our whole, integrated selves—body, mind, soul, and spirit—to our spiritual practice and faith.

For me, there have been two key questions to explore as I have embarked on this integral path:

1. Does engaging the body as a temple of the Holy Spirit help one to fully engage in a personal relationship with God?
2. If "physical" Yoga—*Asana* yoga, or Hatha yoga—was designed to facilitate the understanding and complete mastery of the mind so that practitioners could connect with the divine, is it possible that Christians who engage in the practice of physical yoga and meditation can do so similarly, as preparation to encounter the kingdom of God within?

My own experience responds to these questions with a resounding "yes." And while I know this to be true, I also admit that since the ideas presented in this book might evoke mixed reactions, I write with some fear and trepidation, and also a deep abiding love of God. At times I may offer some viewpoints that you believe to be untrue, and rather than reacting, I invite you to join me in viewing any differences as an opening for a conversation in the true spirit of Christianity as The Episcopal Church understands it. The Episcopal Church determines our theological understanding based on the Anglican path as the "middle way" or *via media*. "The intention of the middle way has been to achieve a comprehensiveness or breadth of approach that could draw wisdom from every side and include the insights of others."[4]

My journey acknowledges that other people and other perspectives have something to teach me—about the world, God, and myself. I am a pilgrim on this journey. I am listening to my teachers both in the church and on the mat, and to my inner teacher, my God, who speaks to me in my heart. I trust in the words of the Psalmist (Psalm 16:7):

> "I bless the Lord who gives me counsel; in the
> night also my heart instructs me."

God continues to speak to my heart as I integrate yoga into my Christian walk. The body is the vehicle in this life through which we encounter the divine. The body is an integral component in this journey called life; without the body, we are simply spirit and consciousness. The journey isn't only about the body, but it certainly doesn't exclude it. The heart, the mind, the soul, and the spirit, completely full of love and devotion in the Spirit of Christ, seek God with faculties beyond the body—and yet, the body is part of our story, our song, our expression and unique manifestation of our individual soul.

I invite you into a way of following Jesus with your whole self—*body, mind, soul, and spirit*—on and off the mat. The yogic path to fully awaken and live is resonant with the Christian path of devotion and service, following Christ and seeking the kingdom of God. May it be for each of us just as Jesus promised:

*"Behold, the kingdom of God is within you"* (Luke 17:21, KJV).

When we look earnestly and humbly within, what truth do we find? We find the eyes to see and the ears to hear the divine truth within us. We find God. But please don't take my word for it; this is a discovery you'll have to make yourself. My desire and honor is to help you find your way.

# ~1~

# The Birthing of YogaMass –
## *Creativity and Courage*

*The only unique contribution that we will ever make
in this world will be born of our creativity.*
*—Dr. Brené Brown, The Daring Way™*

## The Dawn of a New Era

Picture a gathering of people from all across the country, toting water bottles and camping chairs, backpacks, and notepads with pens all over the campground. This isn't just any campground. This was the first annual Wild Goose Festival, in the great, beautiful outdoors of North Carolina. It was 2011, and since I had been too young to experience Woodstock, I was ecstatic to discover that it was a Woodstock sort of gathering: peace, love, and Jesus, without illegal street drugs and overdoses. Young adults with dreadlocks and tattoos, children running and playing and creating art, musicians with guitars and tablas and sitars, singers, authors, theologians, pastors, middle-age seekers, and old hippies still dreaming of a world of peace and non-violence, all gathered in the countryside to celebrate Jesus and the wild goose, which symbolizes the Holy Spirit in Celtic spirituality. A real Jesus "love fest!" I had been waiting for this all my life, an experience of heaven on earth.

It was the first gathering of its kind in the United States, organized by Jim Wallis of Sojourners Magazine and modeled on the Greenbelt gatherings in the U.K. Was American Christianity ready for it? Emphatically, yes. It was a love fest of over 2,000 people gathered in the tent revival mode of sharing the Good News and talking about our faith in creative ways not often expressed in church. It was at Wild Goose that I discovered a rekindling of my faith in my body outside of my yoga practice: I used my body to walk from tent to tent, I got hot, then thirsty, I ate and I drank, and collectively, all of us gathered shared the same space with our bodies and a hunger for this particular kind of faith-filled thinking. I waved blue ribbons as Shane Claiborne, the founder of The Simple Way in Philadelphia and a leading figure in the New Monastic movement, described his journey into Afghanistan with other activists at the start of the "shock and awe" military campaign. His film crew captured the Wild Goose Festival crowd as we sang old-time hymns for the people of Afghanistan with whom he wanted to share an important message: that some people in the United States actually cared about them. This was faith in action, and my heart and soul wept tears that I hadn't felt in a long time as I sat in the midst of a community of faith.

Phyllis Tickle, the late American writer, poet, book publisher and journalist addressing religion and spiritual issues, gave a talk at the Festival about the "Great Emergence." She described the 500-hundred year cycle of Christianity (and Judaism) that results in a "generalized social/political/economic/ intellectual/cultural shift."[5] On either side of the pivotal point is a 100-year period of increasing change to the status quo, the pivotal "event," and then a 50–60 year transition period until the new normal settles in. The advent of secularized Christianity in the US in the last century and the propensity of many to declare that they are "spiritual but not religious," are clear indications of a "new normal" settling in. My own spiritual journey had made many twists and turns and most significantly was impacted by my meditation practice over the years, with a rising sense of wonder at my spiritual awakening happening through my yoga practice, which was giving me an even deeper sense of touching the divine than I had ever experienced. If I was experiencing transition into a new normal, I could only surmise others were too.

In examining the 500-year transformation cycle of the church, we gain an understanding of the shifts occurring right now—the underlying dismantling of traditional forms of faith community and worship—and we gain a perspective on how we might make sense of it all. It is natural that when the status quo is challenged, we feel unsettled. Tickle reminds us it's not our fault. It's the cycle, and we are in it. I choose to see the shifts taking place as an opportunity rather than a threat, as I embrace the promise from the one seated on the throne: "See, I am making all things new" (Revelation 21:5).

## The Great Emergence

The 500-year cycles are not exact on the year; nonetheless, they offer a big picture perspective that is informative and can be exciting. The Great Transformation of the 6th century with "the work of Gregory the Great...and the reconfigured form of Western monasticism, functioned not only as a way of private holiness but also as a way of societal and political stability."[6] About 500 years later, in the 11th century, the Great Schism occurred whereby Rome severed itself from Eastern and Orthodox Christianity to establish its absolute theological or ecclesial authority. That must have been a very unsettling time for Christians.

Again, about 500 years later in the 16th century, the Great Reformation; after a century of cultural pressures and the desire of the faithful to see reform in the Roman church, Martin Luther tacked his 95 theses to the door of the church at Wittenberg Castle in Germany. It was the year 1517, and it marked the beginning of the Great Reformation "characterized by the rise of capitalism, of the middle class, of the nation-state, and finally of Protestantism."[7]

In the years that followed, the printing press allowed the printing and distribution of Holy Scripture, prayer books, and hymnals (in various languages, including English) that inevitably had great significance in the life of the people. No longer were the Bibles and Prayer Books only available to bishops, clergy, and monastics as they had been. The Holy Spirit was placing the tools of the faith directly in the hands of the people. A shift in consciousness at the individual level was clearly beginning with that great transition.

At the turn of the 20th century, social, political, cultural, and theological shifts were well underway. In 1859, Darwin's *The Origin of Species* was published outlining his theory of evolution. In the early 19th century, Sigmund Freud introduced conscious and unconscious states of being, although they could be found in Vedic literature from millennia of old.[8] Carl Jung, Swiss psychiatrist and psychotherapist in the 20th century expanded on Freud's work, opening up the realm of the collective unconscious for exploration and study.

With the advent of radio and television, thinkers and experimenters, and many scholars, pushed our society further into the interior, causing us to question the old, standing definitions of self as they had been given to us. Then came Buddhism with all the tools needed to enter the subjective experience fully and fearlessly...fully, fearlessly, and unencumbered by theism.[9] This marked new challenges for religious institutions in which theism is the foundational component of their faith, the belief in God. The word "theism" originates from the Greek word *Theos,* which means "god." Theism is the belief in the existence of a god or gods, specifically of a creator who intervenes in the universe.

The church had lost the contemplative practices with the rise of the scientific mind, and these practices were beginning to flourish again in the twentieth century after a rediscovery, thanks to spiritual fathers such as Thomas Merton, Thomas Keating, Laurence Freeman, Bede Griffiths, and others. In the deepest gratitude, these brave and bold church fathers were re-introducing the monastic spiritual practices of our Christian tradition from the earliest centuries as well as beginning a practice of interfaith dialogue to learn of the spiritual experiences and expertise of other religious traditions, including our Asian neighbors. The drug age of the 1960s and '70s, in spite of the broken hearts and lives it damaged, provided a new and different understanding of reality. The world-wide-web and the Internet allowed for faster and faster communication and connection with people around the globe. The foundational question of all human existence, according to Phyllis Tickle, arose again with these changes: "Where now is the authority?"[10]

This shift of the 16th century and beyond has led to where we are now, and understanding the larger cycles allows me to feel hopeful that God is doing something new again, as unsettling as it may seem to many. YogaMass is an expression of that newness, just as emergent church expressions and varied forms of new music are changing worship experiences in many churches. Church and pipe organs and hymns from of old are still revered, yet now there are many more options of worship expressions. In the last forty years or so, worship styles have changed to provide different expressions of music and prayer styles: electric guitars and drums, artists painting and sculpting as expression of what they are hearing and feeling during worship services, and big screen projections of sermon illustrations and lyrics to the new praise songs. Even women's ordinations and feminine voices from the pulpit in some Christian denominations are providing new perspectives on the teachings of Jesus!

Tickle articulates the defining moment of the Great Emergence, the term she uses for the 500-year shift that is happening now and began around the turn of the 20th century, with the tragic American event that we know as 9/11. It was a time when everything shifted; everything as we knew it changed and *we* were forever changed. We all remember what we were doing that fateful morning when we first heard the news. Time stood still, and we were changed as a country and as a global society. For Christians in particular, this Great Emergence has left us with two complementary questions, as Tickle defines them:

1. What is human consciousness and/or the humanness of the human?
2. What is the relation of all religions to one another— or, how can we live responsibly as devout and faithful adherents of one religion in a world of many religions?[11]

These are the questions of our time, while we are in the transition to what will become. The question of human consciousness is expressed globally for the spiritual seeker via social media and online seminars. Human consciousness, it seems to me, relates specifically to the science of the mind as addressed by yogic philosophy. As someone who is passionate about interfaith dialogue and the baptismal vow in The Episcopal Church that "I will strive for justice and peace among all people, and respect the dignity of every human being," the second question speaks to the relationships we have with all people, and it is a relevant question in today's pluralistic, global society.

As I ponder these two questions, I have discovered that my responses arise most clearly when I am deep in meditation or intentionally practicing on my yoga mat. That is when my heart sings silently in its depths, for myself, for others, and for all of God's people. In the depth of that silence, my heart invites, "Thy kingdom come, thy will be done."

## Following My Heart

In the Prologue of *The Rule of Benedict* written in the 6th Century, Saint Benedict says, "Listen carefully, my child, to my instructions, and attend to them with the ear of your heart."[12]

It began the way God always works with me—as a persistent nudge that I am supposed to do something, to do this. What I was intuiting was that I was to create a new way of worshipping God with an integration of what I love—my passion, my heart, my inspiration.

My heart was speaking loudly to me, just as it had over my lifetime. The question was, once again, was I listening, and how would I respond? When I offer spiritual direction, and my directee is struggling and experiencing confusion and chaos, I often ask, "What does your heart say?" Now I was asking myself this question.

As a young child, I always wanted to be a mother. It was instinctual I suppose, as it is for many women. In my "School Days" journal that my mother gave me, I wrote as a preschooler that I wanted to be a mom. There it was: my deepest dream was simply to be a mom. And then my aspirations grew after Neil Armstrong was the first man to ever walk on the moon: now I wanted to be an astronaut! How exciting to venture out into space, to discover something altogether new, and to set out on an adventure of a lifetime. Clearly I had an adventurous soul from my earliest years. How interesting that my soul wanted to experience the vastness of the universe at such an early age. Although I didn't have the awareness or the language for it yet, I believe now this yearning was less about science and more about the mystical life. (Awareness, as I am using it in this book, is a state of consciousness, a state of understanding, of having knowledge.)

And then my journal reflected again for the next few years that I wanted to be a mother. It would be almost 25 years later before I would become a mother, and I am grateful every day for the gift and privilege from God to have raised a son who is strong, inner-directed, kind, compassionate, loving, and wise beyond his years.

Life has a way of bringing things full circle—perhaps not exactly as we hope for—and in retrospect, we can see that life brings to us the people, the experiences, the circumstances that teach us what we need to learn.

When I was 17 years old, I heard my calling into ministry. I was sitting outside the apartment complex waiting for my friend Cathy. It was a typical summer night in South Texas: the stars were out in full blaze, and it was balmy and humid with a clear and starry night sky. I sat under the stars, looking into the vastness—which always makes me think of the Creator God— quiet and reflective. I suddenly and unexpectedly heard a voice in my heart speak very clearly and loudly: "Become a priest." I literally laughed out loud, just as Abraham's wife, Sarah, did when she heard she would become pregnant as an older woman well beyond child-bearing years.

It's not so easy to admit you laughed at God. I just couldn't even imagine giving my life completely over to God and going into ministry. I only attended church sporadically and was not active in a faith community. I don't know where my friend and I were headed that night, but I know it wasn't church. Yet when I occasionally attended service, the church brought me solace and peace. I would slip in quietly to experience the deep mystery of Holy Eucharist on Sunday mornings in the little Episcopal Church in my hometown of Kingsville, Texas. There were periodic rare Sundays when I awoke knowing deep down that my very life depended on my getting up and going to church. I didn't understand it, but I knew it to be true; it was God beckoning me home, drawing me into the embrace of the Spirit. I sensed a deep inner knowing that ultimately it was just God and me. On those rare mornings, I watched silently and intently as the Priest celebrated the Eucharist, and the mystery would bring me to tears.

That's why I love the Episcopal Church. The mystery of the real presence of Christ in the Eucharist is celebrated, revered, and upheld in an ongoing tradition with the lineage back to the very beginning, to those who walked with Jesus.

It was during that same time in my life that I practiced yoga with the PBS yoga teacher. I was mesmerized and deeply happy while doing the practice; my heart sang when she guided her viewers through a thirty-minute series of *asanas* (yoga poses) and then *Savasana* (relaxation in "Corpse Pose.") I couldn't wait until the show was on again, and I faithfully followed her class every week. I didn't have a yoga mat, so I practiced on a floor rug we had in our den. What she was doing made me feel good: relaxed, balanced, strong—the qualities that cultivate inner peace. This was as important for me then as it is now: I liked the way yoga made me *feel*. At that time, I really needed this new discovery. I had made choices that left me in spiritual deprivation and physical dis-ease. I was living on the edge in smoke-filled coliseum halls of rock concerts and nightclubs teeming with light shows, smoke, tequila sours, and loud, energizing dance music.

Then I left home for college in Austin at The University of Texas, and the college budgets, big city lights, and stimulating academic university setting took precedence, and my lifestyle turned serious in study and part-time work. Practicing yoga fell by the wayside. Attending church wasn't a draw for me or for my friends. With God's help—in a miraculous way—even without yoga and without a faith community, I left behind the self-destructive lifestyle that was damaging my body and my soul. Not completely, but I was on my way to recovery and healing. God was leading me to new life, as much of a struggle as it was, in spite of myself. God was always there for me, even when I had strayed far, far away.

Slowly, I felt empowered to begin again.

## Birthing Creativity (Speaking My Truth)

Almost three decades later, God planted another seed in me, and my spiritual awakening began to open, slowly, and with lots of turns on the winding path. Wise yogis teach, "It takes as long as it takes." My life's path unfolded in ordinary and not-so-ordinary ways. Marriage. Pregnancy. Widowhood. Motherhood. Second Marriage. Meditation. Spiritual director commissioning. Seminary. Yoga. Benedictine Oblate vows. Ordination to the Priesthood. Spiritual leadership. Sermons. Pastoral care. Yoga. Yoga teacher training. YogaMass.

I discovered in my 30s the practice of meditation, sometimes called *contemplative prayer* or centering prayer. The gift of meditation is that it brings you to a place of stillness where you listen to God in the depths of the heart. Meditation allows you to listen for the still, small voice of God in the silence. That still, small voice brought back to me, 20 years later, those same words in the depth of my heart: "Become a priest." This time I recognized it, and I didn't laugh. I moved very slowly, pondering this inner knowing in my heart, for several years, and finally succumbed to an inner calling that only would bring me peace once I started down the path.

It was time to get on with the work I came here to do. God was calling me to open my heart to a new way of being in the world, into a life of service in my own unique way. Creativity is the product of co-creating with God: it has the potential of changing the world and those around you, and it also nurtures your very soul in the process. It was time for me to say yes to co-creating with God through a vocation of ministry with my heart's desire to bring healing into the world.

On my journey to follow the vocation that I was meant to follow, even with circuitous turns, I encountered on a deeper level the spirituality of Mother Mary and Mary Magdalene. Mother Mary inspires me; I am also deeply inspired by Mary Magdalene.

*I wonder, what would have happened if Mother Mary had not said yes to the Angel Gabriel when he brought her the news that she would conceive in her womb and bear a son?* What would my life be like had I not said yes to a *second* call to the priesthood?

Now, God has planted another seed in me, which has brought me full circle into birthing pains. God surprises me, again and again, with unfailing mercy and steadfast love, abounding grace in action. What would happen if now I did not say yes to the calling to bring forth YogaMass, an integrated spirituality and worship experience that honors the transcendent divine and the immanent incarnate divine in you and me? I discerned that I could not *not* dare to be bold and to bring the good news of Christ and his consciousness to those who find themselves on their yoga mats.

Being true to myself and to the movement of God in my heart has been difficult for me as an adult, feeling the need to be responsible and to fulfill expectations (my own and others). I have tended to put others first, acting out of a twisted sort of humility that really was grounded in a lack of self-worth. The practice of self-compassion is much harder for me than offering compassion for others. This is true of many, many, many of us—mostly women, although we wish it weren't so.

Self-compassion begins with listening to my heart and acknowledging what I am feeling. As a teenager, I numbed my feelings. After my first husband died, the sad truth is that I didn't even now how I felt, other than sadness. I couldn't feel anything *but* sadness. That no longer works for me. I want to feel my feelings completely, whether joyful or painful, and give voice to them, and to who I am. Birthing something new from my inner creativity and voice is what my heart deeply desires, as I offer myself to the world in the unique way only I can offer.

Each of us has a unique purpose in our life, and our work is to find that special thing, that unique offering that will make the world a better place. It is the ultimate spiritual practice of following your heart, letting your heart sing. When I celebrate the Eucharist, I am affirmed in my deepest being that I am called to be a priest. My heart sings and my whole being engages in the words and the liturgical movements. When I share the gospel so that others will know they are loved completely, thoroughly, unconditionally, and forever, I find deep gladness. God's grace trumps missing the mark, the true definition of sin. Love wins. Always. My story proves it, again and again.

When I'm on my yoga mat, my soul and body surrender to what is. The movements and the breath work bring me to a point of intentional focus on the "here and now," the present moment, so that my mind slows down its normal chatter. I let go of the thoughts and feelings I brought with me, and for this moment in time, I'm focused on *this* breath, *this* stretch, *this* contraction, *this* expansion, *this* pose. Every part of me becomes part of a fluid movement of body and soul, breath and energy. *What is* at this moment is all there is, and my body releases the repressed emotions that no longer serve me. My body becomes the vehicle for surrender into my life as it is—not as I wish it to be, but as it is: beautiful, broken, and blessed.

The birthing of YogaMass took time, as does any gestation process. But that time is God's time, "Kairos" (καιρός) time in Greek. We can't rush God's time. We can only surrender to the process and allow it to unfold, as God would have it unfold. Life for me has had a distinct direction and purpose, as Dr. Brené Brown describes in her book, *I Thought it Was Just Me*: "As long as we're creating, we're cultivating meaning." I have been following God's lead to integrate what I have learned and to open the experience for others.

In December 2015, with an intimate group of friends from Grace Episcopal Church, Houston, where I serve as the Vicar, and the Institute for Spiritualty and Health, we had a dry run of YogaMass. It was a beautiful and grace-filled experience. We practiced the music, the flow, and the logistics. We set the lighting, the ambience, the incense. We offered our first public YogaMass on January 30, 2016.

One of the participants in our first ever YogaMass was overheard saying, "This is the first sermon I didn't fall asleep to!" Actually, we didn't offer a formal sermon at that first YogaMass. I simply led guided reflections on the gospel reading while we moved to hatha flow with our bodies and our breath. It's hard to fall asleep when you're up on your mat and moving!

The birth of YogaMass had come, gracefully and perfectly, just as God's timing is always perfect. Aligning with the consciousness of Christ and the movement of the Spirit always brings perfection, not the kind of obsessive perfection that drives us to strive to be good enough until we make ourselves sick, but the kind of simple and graceful perfection that allows space for imagination and creativity to percolate, and gently brings the new creation into reality in perfect timing. "Be perfect, therefore, as your heavenly Father is perfect" (Matthew 5:48). All in God's time, in God's way—not forced but simply allowed. It is grace upon grace.

## Birthing Courage

I am grateful to Bishop C. Andrew Doyle, IX Bishop of the Episcopal Diocese of Texas, for many things, and particularly for his support of my vision and the creation of YogaMass, for allowing me to step out in faith and offer this type of service. Bishop Doyle is imaginative, creative, and bold, and his spiritual leadership makes room for unique ways of worship. YogaMass is a non-traditional worship service: new, different, and innovative. I'm grateful for his encouragement and his acknowledgment that it might be a hard road for me, and that I need to be prepared to face my critics. I trust that everything will unfold in God's time and that I was, in fact, being prepared for living courageously in the face of both criticism and affirmation.

All in God's time, Bishop Doyle brought Dr. Brené Brown, research professor at the University of Houston Graduate College of Social Work and author of *The Gifts of Imperfection, I Thought It Was Just Me,* and *Daring Greatly* to clergy in the diocese for a week-long immersion in The Daring Way™. The Daring Way™ teaches wholehearted living and daring greatly as we live our lives and follow our hearts. It helps to provide context for our feelings of shame and vulnerability when we are stepping out into the unknown. This process is so resonant with the gospel when Jesus teaches us, "Do not be afraid."

I knew I would be going for Yoga teacher training that summer, and I knew that adventure would lead me deeper into my heart and my calling. How important and perfect was God's timing to help me experience what courage felt like so that I could prepare to live into the nudgings in my heart.

It takes courage to step into the unknown and try something new for you. It takes the courage to fail and to try again, or try it differently. Dr. Brown understands how unsettling it is to step out into the unknown:

> "You can chose courage or comfort, but you cannot have both." (The Daring Way™)

It takes a good sense of grounding to accept that you might fail, and it will be okay. We all try, we make mistakes, we fail, and the hope is that we can get back up and keep on trying. Sometimes we have to modify the course and change our plans. But living life is all in the journey, not in the future "end goal." To live is to engage— to engage with our dreams, our hearts, each other, our neighbors, and God. So it does come down to courage. How willing am I to fully engage with life, with my heart, with God?

I needed this kind of courage to step beyond the traditional role of priest and become a yoga educator. I believe that God places events, circumstances, and people on our path right when they're supposed to happen, and exactly at the right time. I prayed for courage to request approval to offer the YogaMass liturgy and experience at Grace Episcopal Church in Houston where I serve as Vicar. I even wondered if this might be the end of my priesthood since this integration of yoga and the Eucharist was non-traditional, much different than our authorized liturgies in the *Book of Common Prayer*. Much to my surprise, Bishop Andy Doyle graciously accepted my proposal with his imaginative and creative spirit. He is open to trying new ways to be the missional church so that more people will hear the good news of the gospel of Jesus Christ. This is how YogaMass was birthed, with a sprinkling of creativity, imagination, courage, faith, and unbridled determination.

One of my favorite yoga teachers in Austin, Texas, beautiful Camilla, says, "It is more courageous to feel life than it is to think life." We have two options for "feeling" life. Option one is that we can stay stuck in the past and focus only on what happened before, and allow our feelings and energy around past events to remain stuck in our minds and bodies. But if we allow those feelings to stay repressed without expression, they can do physical, emotional or even spiritual harm to ourselves and to others.

Or, we have a second option: we can use those feelings and passions to create energy for movement and momentum, so that we always keep moving forward. It is a choice. Sometimes the bravest thing we can do is to keep living (a line I heard in a cowboy movie)! The only thing we really have to lose by moving forward into our creative and higher self, however, is a life unlived to its fullest potential.

## Living and Giving with all My Heart

It takes inspiration to dream and courage to live our dreams. The older and wiser I become, the more I am willing to rise up out of my fear, doubt, and negative thinking to where my heart is leading me. I have to remind myself to intentionally remember my call to ministry: healing, transformation, and helping others (and myself) find God. How this calling will continue to unfold in my life is a mystery now, as I cannot see too far ahead. But what I do know is that when I engage life, relationships, and myself with all my heart, living in the way my heart is leading me, I feel as though I am being true to myself. My heart leads me as God's Spirit leads me, so when I am following that flow, I know I am also being true to God. This is true peace. Flow is my personal mantra. I pray to be in the flow: to be present to it, to flow with it without fear and without resistance, simply gracefully riding that wave of life energy that is me and all of creation around me.

Mary Oliver, the great poet of nature, God, and life outdoors, describes so poignantly the experience of the desire to follow our hearts:

## Everything[13]

I want to make poems that say right out, plainly,
    what I mean, that don't go looking for the
laces of elaboration, puffed sleeves. I want to
    keep close and use often words like
*heavy, heart, joy, soon,* and to cherish
    the question mark and her bold sister

the dash. I want to write with quiet hands. I
    want to write while crossing the fields that are
fresh with daisies and everlasting and the
    ordinary grass. I want to make poems while thinking of
the bread of heaven and the
    cup of astonishment; let them be

songs in which nothing is neglected,
    not a hope, not a promise. I want to make poems
that look into the earth and the heavens
    and see the unseeable. I want them to honor
both the heart of faith, and the light of the world;
    the gladness that says, without any words, *everything.*

Following our hearts into the heart of God is the spiritual journey. As we listen to our hearts, our spirits connect with Spirit, to the sacredness among us and within us. We birth what God wishes to say and do through us, that which is our unique voice in the evolution of humanity.

# 2

# Engaging Aliveness –
## *Being Fully Human*

> The miracle isn't walking on water but walking
> on the earth, fully alive to every moment.
> –*Thich Nhat Hanh, Wholeness: Blessed are the Peacemakers*

Setting aside time for soul connection is a direct way of experiencing God and seeing with new eyes. I love this story of an American traveler on safari in Kenya that so beautifully illustrates the importance of sacred time. He was loaded down with maps, and timetables, and travel agendas. Porters from a local tribe were carrying his cumbersome supplies, luggage, and "essential stuff." On the first morning, everyone awoke early and traveled fast and went far into the bush. On the second morning, they all woke very early and traveled very fast and went very far into the bush. On the third morning, they all woke very early and traveled very fast and went even farther into the bush. The American was pleased. But on the fourth morning, the porters refused to move. They simply sat by a tree. Their behavior incensed the American. "This is a waste of valuable time. Can someone tell me what is going on here?" The translator answered, "They are waiting for their souls to catch up with their bodies."

In our ordinary, daily lives, we often take for granted that we are breathing, that we are alive. We go about our days fulfilling checklists, doing what needs to be done, and interacting with others in all kinds of relationships. We engage with ourselves only when we take time to listen inwardly to our own needs and desires. We search for happiness, we search for experiences that feed our souls, and we search for fulfilling relationships. A good spiritual practice is to reflect on what or whom we choose to engage with. Do we search for God? Do we engage with life, fully and wholeheartedly? Do we engage with the sacred? Do we engage and interact with the experience of being alive in this body, celebrating that we are an embodied spiritual being?

Engaging aliveness is experiencing the gift of being fully alive. It is consciousness or clear awareness of the sacredness of everything. Engaging aliveness is a spiritual practice, and it includes sacred time, space, breath, and energy.

## The Body in Sacred Time

When you hear the phrase "Be here now," coined by Ram Dass, the American spiritual teacher and author, do you think of the body? Or do you think of this term as referring only to a psychological or spiritual state? Does the mind think of slowing itself, moving into a meditative state, having a higher state of consciousness? Surely it is about the mind, but it is also about the body, and it is about the soul. It is about being in a state of awareness of sacred time, of holy time, of eternity, now.

Often it is hard for we busy people to slow down and savor the present moment. In our fast-paced culture, with too many demands and too many messages flashing on our smart phones calling for our attention, it becomes essential that we make time for nurturing our spiritual lives. People everywhere, across all faith traditions, are increasingly hungry for "soul time" that allows the soul to breathe and relax. Finding time for the soul to breathe is essential to our health and well-being, individually and as a society. We have lost that connection over these last few centuries but the connection is thankfully being re-established through contemplative practices in Christianity and across many faith traditions. Some find "soul time" in worship, others in nature, others in yoga studios, others in their private devotional and spiritual time at home.

In Judeo-Christian terms, God gifted us with Sabbath to give us time to reconnect with our souls and with God. The traditional Jewish Sabbath begins Friday at sundown, the Christian Sabbath with Sunday morning worship. In both, Sabbath time begins with the lighting of candles (Christians light our candles at the altar of the Lord's table) and a stopping—to welcome the Sabbath in. In this sacred time, we try to be attuned to the holiness of time and to God's nearest presence. Jewish writer Marcia Falk, in Wayne Buller's book *Sabbath: Finding Rest, Renewal, and Delight in our Busy Lives,* tells of her experience of the Sabbath: *"Three generations back my family had only to light a candle and the world parted. Today, Friday afternoon, I disconnect clocks and phones. When night fills my house with passages, I begin saving my life."*[14]

Awakening to a clear awareness of God's presence in sacred time is the gift the church can give us. Taking sacred time in the form of the Sabbath is the time for bringing the true essence of eternity into the now. This is the time for finding life, engaging life, and for saving life. We can set aside sacred time for meditation, contemplative prayer, devotional prayers, and for a yoga practice, any time. I like to describe my twenty minutes of meditation twice a day as mini-Sabbath time. We can set aside sacred time for worship in a community to experience the eternal now together.

Joan Chittister, Order of St. Benedict (O.S.B.), speaks to the spiritual question, "Is there life after death?" when she relays this story: "A disciple once asked a Holy One this question, who answered, 'The great spiritual question of life is not, *Is there life after death? The great spiritual question is, Is there life before death?'"*[15]

When we awaken to life in its true essence, we awaken to a clear awareness that life is now. Not later. Now. In this present moment.

## Sacred Space

Awakening to an awareness of the divine makes the ordinary simply remarkable and extraordinary. Being becomes a gift, an art, an expression. Often we need guideposts to help us on the path to clear awareness, a higher consciousness, and we call these spiritual disciplines. Spiritual disciplines are just what they say they are: disciplines. Many think of discipline as something punitive, or restricting, a form of keeping society or one's self "in check." Spiritual disciplines do help us maintain a sense of stability, for the simple purpose of staying focused on the desire to experience God and the sacredness of it all.

Once you begin on the spiritual path, finding or creating the space to stay true to the practice is essential to the spiritual life. Making a commitment to a spiritual discipline or disciplines is the first step, and it is so much easier to continue it if there is place where you can go, be it a park, a yoga studio, a church, or a dedicated space in your home or outdoor space to practice it. Some set aside a whole room in their home for prayer, meditation and yoga—others, like myself, can't help utilizing the whole house for different aspects of our spiritual disciplines!

Creating dedicated, intentional space that draws you into your spiritual practices helps you to keep up the discipline of being attentive to your spiritual life. In the church, we intentionally use different elements to create sacred space, such as candles, incense, and crosses, and it is the ongoing, collective worship, filled with soulful music that makes you feel alive and grateful to God, along with the prayers of the people, that deepen the space and invite God's Holy Spirit in for a divine encounter with God.

A yoga studio intentionally focused on the spiritual life will also have elements that create sacred space. It may include calm colors, the smell of sweet incense from India, or a statue of the Buddha or a wall hanging with the Buddha's calm, serene face. Peaceful music sweetly caresses you to slow down, relax, and center into yourself. Creating a peaceful space that allows you to settle onto your mat and into your body allows for the gentle touching of the heart and soul.

## The Zen Understanding of Space

I happily tagged along with a friend on a business trip to Tokyo a few years ago, and we decided to visit Kyoto, Japan, to learn more of its deep history and view the beautiful monasteries reflecting splendor, simplicity, and serenity. The Zen monasteries and gardens were breathtaking. It was late fall and peak season for cherry blossom trees. This South Texas girl had never seen such incredible beauty, not just in nature, but also in the landscaping. There was a simplicity that soothes the soul. There was space that allowed the soul to breathe, to wonder, to sing. I watched young lovers stroll through the peaceful gardens, and occasionally they would stop and embrace, absorbing the peaceful energy into their beings and their relationship.

The well-defined walkways with pea gravel and rock borders invite you into the garden. Many of the gardens have sand spaces that are raked perfectly smooth, with circular patterns marked in them to draw your eyes into the feminine, circular movement of infinity. Carefully placed foliage, trees, and bushes surrounded serene ponds or lakes that gave off a reflection of its peaceful surroundings. My favorite image, and the one that lingered the longest, was the Zen Buddhist temple in Kyoto: the Temple of the Golden Pavilion at Kinkaku-ji. The day we visited, the Temple was adorned with a clear blue sky, and the still lake gracefully embodied the temple and the sky, mirroring it back, forming a complete union with it. Yin and yang, matter and water, mirror and reflection—not two, distinct and separate, but two dancing with each other, two inseparable and flowing into one.

Whether you are called to peaceful space for meditation, prayer, yoga or your very life, finding or creating that space is nurturing and life giving. Forming space for yourself and others that engages the senses and draws you deeper into the heart makes room for reflection and rest, centering and breathing. I do not know who to credit this quote to, but I love it: "This is your space...where all the noise of your life ceases to exist. For as long as you are in this space, you are untouchable." That is the goal of creating a sacred space where you can go and find your center. It is a gift to yourself.

## The Body As a Sacred Vessel

Experiencing the body as a vessel of sacred space seems foreign to many people. The Tibetan Buddhists have a meditation that imagines your body as being hollow. It is a wonderful way to relax and feel the vastness of space within you:

> *Beginning the guided meditation in the head, imagine that there is clear space behind your eyes, in your brain, behind your nose, behind your ears, and into your neck.*

> *The space may be filled with clear, cool blue sky.*

> *As you travel down your body—arms, hands, chest, abdomen, back, pelvis, legs, feet, toes—imagine clear blue sky filling you completely.*

Sometimes I like to imagine warm light filling that space as I move back up the body in the reverse direction. This sweet meditation is a beautiful way for me to relax the body and be comfortable in my own skin, my own container.

Here is another meditation in which you may also experience your body in a sacred way:

*Sit in a comfortable meditation position.*

*To feel your body, inhale slowly. Then exhale slowly.*

*Long, slow inhalations, followed by even longer, slower exhalations slow you down and help you focus on the gift of breath.*

*During the breaths, pay attention to what you experience, what you are sensing in your body.*

*Does the body hurt, and where?*

*Can you breathe into the belly, the ribs, the chest, and then exhale chest, ribs, belly?*

*What does it feel like to experience the breath in the front of the ribs, and the back and side ribs? What does it feel like to breathe into the back body, behind the heart?*

*What feelings or memories arise for you?*

Self-inquiry, the practice of inquiring into the experience and feelings of the self, is a beautiful practice illuminated by breathing. It can create peace, increased understanding, and bring new insights. Yet it also may be difficult at times, bringing up emotions and memories that have been tucked away. In that case, let the emotions and memories arise, notice them, and then release them in a way that recognizes them but doesn't allow your mind to pick them up, entertain them, or hold on to them. The breath work provides a way to calm the mind, to slow it down, and to center down into the body and your very being-ness. When I lead meditation groups, I guide participants in long slow inhales and exhales so that we are breathing rhythmically together. As we breathe, we invite the Holy Spirit into our midst, as Jesus promises, "For where two or three are gathered in my name, I am there among them" (Matthew 18:20). As we inhale, we breathe in God's Holy Spirit, and as we exhale, we share our breath with the world around us. Inhale and exhale, receive and let go.

## Sacred Breath

The practice of yogic breath work (or *pranayama* in Sanskrit) is life-giving. Breathing while meditating on God, the eternal source of life, from the heart space opens a whole realm of possibilities of relating to God. In the Christian Holy Scriptures (both the Old and New Testaments), breath is sacred, and breath animates life. To fully understand the meaning of breath in Scripture, we begin with the Greek word *pneuma,* which is air in movement, blowing, breathing out of air. *Pneuma* also means breath, that which animates or gives life to the body (life-spirit). *Pneuma* is used in Luke 23:46:

> "Then Jesus, crying with a loud voice, said, 'Father, into your hands I commend my spirit' (*pneuma*). Having said this, he breathed his last."

*Pneuma* has a similar meaning to the Hebrew word *ruach. Ruach,* in the Tanakh (the primary Jewish Sacred text), generally means "wind," "breath," "mind," or "spirit." In the second verse of the Bible, the word *Ruach Elohim* is used:

> "The earth was a formless void and darkness covered the face of the deep, while a wind from God *(Ruach Elohim,* spirit of *Elohim)* swept over the face of the waters" (Genesis 1:2).

In Hebrew, *Elohim* is the name for God as the Creator and Judge of the universe. Using the Hebrew Interlinear Bible, the translation is even more beautiful and resonant with the energetic vibrations felt in yogic breathing in this translation of the second half of this same verse:

> "...the spirit of *Elohim* vibrating over the waters."

*Ruach* is the breath of both animals and humankind, and God is the creator of *ruach*:

> "As long as my breath is in me and the spirit *(ruach)* of God is in my nostrils" (Job 27:3).

God's *ruach* is the source of life and indicates creative activity and active power:

> "By the word of the Lord the heavens were made, and all their host by the breath *(ruach)* of his mouth" (Psalm 33:6).

The *ruach* of God imparts the divine image to man, and constitutes the animating dynamic which results in humankind's *nephesh* as the self with a personal life. *Nephesh* in the Old Testament Hebrew Lexicon is defined as the soul—the whole, living being of an individual person—and is even more descriptive: self, life, creature, person, appetite, mind, living being, desire, emotion, passion, that which breathes, the breathing substance or being, soul, the inner being of man, the man himself, self, person or individual, the seat of emotions and passions, including activity of the mind and will. It is important to note that the soul includes the mind and will, and mind is not separate from soul.

The breath of God that gives us life also gives each of us a share in God's life, in God's creative Spirit, as our souls open up to a life in God's Spirit. Our spirits—the vital, dynamic forces of being that are given by God and bring our souls (our individuality) into life—are enlivened through our breath. When I first encountered the question in a yoga class, "Are you breathing, or are you being breathed?" I was awestruck to realize that yogic practice intentionally teaches the awareness that breath (Sanskrit *prana*) works "in us," just as the Christian (and Jewish) faith upholds God's life-giving breath (*ruach, pneuma*) within us. When we breathe involuntarily, we are unaware that God's breath is actually breathing us. God (and God's *ruach*) is present with us every single moment of our lives. When we voluntarily breathe with awareness that we are breathing, we are intentionally participating with God, co-creating life itself in this body.

We have evidence of this presence of God's Spirit imparted by Jesus after his resurrection when he appeared to his apostles:

> "Jesus said to them again, 'Peace be with you. As the Father has sent me, so I send you.' When he had said this, he breathed on them and said to them, 'Receive the Holy Spirit'" [*pneuma*] (John 20:21-22).

He was imparting through his breath the Holy Spirit. To experience the breath is to experience God's *ruach,* the Holy Spirit. Recognizing the gift of breath is awareness of the gift of God's life-giving action within us. This is true whenever and wherever we are aware of our breath.

This reminds me of the beautiful hymn in the Episcopal Church's 1982 Hymnal, "Breathe on me, breath of God" by Edwin Hatch, 1878:

> Breathe on me, Breath of God, fill me with life anew,
> that I may love the way you love, and do what you would do.

Breathe on me, Breath of God, until my heart is pure,
until my will is one with yours, to do and to endure.

Breathe on me, Breath of God, so shall I never die,
but live with you the perfect life for all eternity.

*A Simple Meditation*

A simple meditation is to return to the peaceful place inside created by feeling your heartbeat and breathing. The medieval Christian mystic, Hildegard of Bingen, said that everything may be felt as a "feather on the breath of God." One meditation is to focus on the breath and the heartbeat and how it keeps you close to the heartbeat of God.[16]

> *Rhythmically tuning into your breath and your heartbeat, imagine that God is breathing you—that your heartbeat is beating alongside and within God's heartbeat.*
>
> *Allow the pulsating sensations to move through your entire body, making you feel alive in this body.*
>
> *Visualize inhaling into your body God's breath, and on the exhale, allowing God's breath to flow out from you.*

This meditation brings awareness of God's closeness, God's presence, both around and within you. When you begin to feel God's breath in you, sustaining life and health, the separateness of God begins to melt away. The kingdom of God, the life force within you, is closer than you realize.

*Pneuma* (breath, air in movement) and *ruach* (wind, breath, spirit) have a similarity to the "winds" as described in yogic literature. *Prana* in yoga, or *Chi* in Chinese medicine, is the vital energy or life force, which keeps the body alive and healthy. *Prana* nourishes the whole body so that it functions properly, and without it, the body would die. *Prana* pervades the whole body, following flow patterns, or *nadis*, which are responsible for maintaining all individual cellular activity. When *prana* begins to flow, toxins that have accumulated in the body are removed, ensuring health and vitality of the whole body.

In yoga, specific breathing techniques are called *pranayama*. There are many instructive books written on the techniques of *pranayama*, and yoga teachers bring a focus on breathing into a yoga practice. When I lead a flow yoga class, I focus intentionally on the breath throughout the flow and in each pose. When we experience the breath in the body, it is healing and makes us feel alive. Giving attention to the breath brings balance and stability. It calms the mind and the body. It helps to put things in perspective. The mind and the body then have a greater chance of not reacting to external stresses and for healing imbalances and dis-ease. Focusing on breath brings awareness that there is something sacred about life, and it is not to be wasted with frenetic activity or frivolous wandering. This is the breath that gives life, and it is all a gift. The body is the vehicle to experiencing the fullness of life with every single, precious breath. *Asanas*—the physical movements—bring another dimension to health, wholeness, and healing.

## The Body is Integral to the Energy of Spirit

In my opinion, Christianity has lacked acknowledgement of the beauty and sacredness of the human body. The focus has been on Christ's body on the cross, and the Body of Christ, our collective togetherness of a community intentionally serving Christ out in the world. But somewhere along the way, the spiritual life became a higher priority over the physical, and a duality was created: the spirit is good, the body is bad. Western Christianity adopted this stance, and as a result, the religious life has failed to recognize and honor the inherent sacredness of the body. If we are made in the image of God, then our bodies, too, must be beautiful and sacred. The movement of yoga into the West has brought to light this tragic omission within our Christian focus.

As yoga practices are incorporated into one's lifestyle, steadiness and grace of movement develop, as well as ease and health of the body and mind. Through a physical practice of *asanas* (yoga postures), the dormant energy potential of a person is released and experienced as increased confidence in all areas of life. Yoga *asanas* help the body to be relieved of tension, aches, and pains, and allow you to sit comfortably for meditation. Swami Satyananda Saraswati explains the purpose of *asanas* from two yogic perspectives—Raja yoga (the mental science) and Hatha yoga (postures and breath work):

> *Asanas* are practiced to develop the ability to sit comfortably in one position for an extended period of time, an ability necessary for meditation. Raja yoga equates *yogasana* to the stable sitting position.

> The hatha yogis, however, found that certain specific body positions, or asanas, open the energy channels and psychic centres. They found that developing control of the body through these practices enabled them to control the mind and energy. *Yogasanas* became tools to higher awareness, providing the stable foundation necessary for exploration of the body, breath, mind and higher states.[17]

The body, then, is a vehicle for us to learn more about ourselves—and even to take us to higher states of consciousness. At times, self-exploration and self-inquiry come by means of silent meditation with a mantra, and at other times, the journey of exploration is amplified when standing in a Warrior pose, counting long, slow breaths, and witnessing the mind's resistance to intentional steadiness when discomfort arises.

Self-inquiry through the body is increasingly becoming a spiritual path for many, as Carolyn Myss, author, speaker, and medical intuitive, describes:

> Today, many spiritual seekers are trying to infuse their daily lives with a heightened consciousness of the sacred, striving to act as if each of their attitudes expressed their spiritual essence. Such conscious living is an invocation, a request for personal spiritual authority. It represents a dismantling of the old religions' classic parent-child relationship to God and a move into spiritual adulthood. Spiritual maturation includes not only developing the ability to interpret the deeper messages of the sacred texts, but learning to read the spiritual language of the body....As spiritual adults we accept responsibility for co-creating our lives and our health.[18]

She goes on to explain the significance of our gradual transformation into conscious spiritual adults:

> "Again and again the sacred texts tell us that our life's purpose is to understand and develop the power of our spirit, power that is vital to our mental and physical well-being."[19]

Applying an understanding of an integrated body, mind, soul, and spirit strengthens our well-being. Body, mind, soul, and spirit are inter-connected and inseparable. Strength or weakness in one affects the others. Approaching the mat with an understanding of the vital energy or life force flowing through your body awakens you to the spirit, God's divine spark, within you. This awareness also awakens potential increased life force when the body is given attention as a part of a whole, as a uniquely created human being.

Religion and Western medicine have for too long created a separation of mind, soul, and spirit from the body, which has resulted in dis-ease and fragmented existence of individuals and the collective society. If we value the bodies we are living in, and work toward integrating them back into our whole beings, we create renewed life energy. If the church honors an integrated approach to mind, body, soul, and spirit, deeper healing on the physical, emotional, psychological, and spiritual levels will be possible for the individual and the collective.

When body, mind, and heart (the seat of the soul) are working together, we can also experience a breakthrough to a new sense of creativity in our life. The body cannot be separated from the mind or the heart. Author Neil Douglas-Klotz describes a series of body prayers that help us focus on the integrated whole of our being:

> While walking, breathe and move together in rhythm. Feel yourself as if drawn from the heart toward a goal or person you love. Try actually moving *from the heart* and notice the effect. At first, make sure you have enough room to move without being interrupted. With some practice, this body prayer can also be used in the crowd to help fortify one's feeling and refocus one's intention.

When in need of healing or rest, or in emotional turmoil, return to the heart-shrine. Let whatever feelings emerge be embraced and acknowledged by the breath of God in your own breathing. Gradually allow the breathing to become more rhythmic. Inhale from the One Source of healing; exhale to that part of yourself in need or turmoil.[20]

Breathing while meditating on God from the heart space opens a whole realm of possibilities of relating to God. Now it gets more real, more personal, more intimate. Yogis teach that the heart space is the center of one's being. Finding God there anchors one into the vastness of God but in a very personal way. It is discovered interiorly, and is sublimely Christian when it is shared in community. Thus, the worship experience must allow for the body and the heart to participate in worship, and for the heart to experience and express what it discovers to be true.

## Awareness of All That Resonates

When two hearts meet and you have a sense that you have known that person for a long, long time, you feel a sense of "knowing" at a level beyond sensory communication. In the best case, you feel a sense of ease and comfort, an inner knowing that all will be well. Sometimes, you may feel a dissonance that you cannot explain. This communication occurs on an energetic or spiritual level; I call it intuition. Intuition helps us know at an energetic or subtle level when an encounter or relationship is healthy or when it may be harmful. Resonating in a positive way with another human being—mind-to-mind, heart-to-heart, and in some cases, body-to-body—is sacred communication, always giving us an opportunity for spiritual or emotional growth. Relationships may be at one or more levels: physical, intellectual, emotional, spiritual, or energetic. At the energetic level, it involves all of our layers of being. When you find your soul mate, you connect at the energetic or subtle body level, which is at the level of "light, energy, emotional feelings, and fluid and flowing images,"[21] as defined by Ken Wilber, author and philosopher.

Communication at the subtle body level creates an energetic feeling of well-being. When I was writing this book, I had one of these experiences I call a "God moment." A friend, Dr. Hansa Medley, named Bhakti (meaning "devotional worship" in Sanskrit), invited me to meet one of her teachers of the International Society for Krishna Consciousness (ISKCON) community in Houston—the Swami who inspired her. She took me to the private home where he was staying, and the three of us met in the living room to meet and talk about my book, about God, and about the path of yoga.

Swami Kesava Bharati Das Goswami spoke of the devotee's desire to be in relationship with the divine, desiring union—not as a merging, but union as a relationship. This is an excellent clarification. We do not "merge" with God, but we "commune" with God. Swami spoke of the love shared, the gift of the exchange between God and the devotee. As he described the exchange between God and the devotee, it reminded me of the Christian doctrine of the Holy Trinity exchanging love between the Father and the Son and the Holy Spirit. Each component of the Trinity equally shares this love and in its abundance, it overflows for the whole world. Swami Kesava Bharati Das Goswami spoke of the highest level of devotion, called *Bhakti* yoga, where you desire this exchange of love so much that you simply cannot stand it another moment. I imagined it to be a desire so overwhelming and all-encompassing that all of one's life becomes completely directed toward the divine.

As Swami spoke to me, with kindness and gentleness, an understanding dawned within me. When he explained that the ultimate goal of yoga is to see God face-to-face, it reminded me of the intensity of the desire of the Christian saints and mystics through the ages to see God and to be in full communion with God at the deepest level. I love Franciscan Friar and spiritual leader Richard Rohr's definition of a mystic: "A mystic is one who has moved from mere belief systems or belonging systems to actual inner experience,"[22]—a spirituality many today can claim.

The saints of the church, the mystics of the Christian faith, and yogis all embody this desire for an inner experience of truth. The word religion comes from the Latin word *religare,* which means, "to bind," classically understood to mean the bond between humans and the divine. *Yoga* in Sanskrit means, "yoke, link, and connect," and is used to signify any form of connection. Dr. Swami Shankardev Saraswati explains that in a philosophical sense, however, *yoga* means the conscious connection of the limited egoic self with the unlimited, eternal, higher Self.

Christians historically haven't been taught to think in terms of our higher Self, but as you will see, the Christian contemplative tradition clearly teaches of the True Self and the False Self (I'll talk more about this in Chapter 4). Christians do desire to enter into the same love bond between the Father, the Son, and the Holy Spirit that Jesus wanted his followers to enter into and experience through him. When we have conversion experiences, they are profound experiences of Jesus' love for us, bringing us into the love of God. As we become more attuned to the higher Self, we become more willing to be absorbed in God's love and to direct our attention toward God and God's action in the world.

Swami Kesava Bharati Das Goswami's description of the devotee's deep desire for an intimate relationship with God resonated with me. I understood what he said from a deep place of knowing, as if I had known it already and he was simply speaking my truth. There we were: two souls resonating heart-to-heart. What he was saying was not really different from the path of loving God "with all your heart, and with all your soul, and with all your strength, and with all your mind," as Jesus taught (Luke 10:27). As I listened and nodded and smiled, he placed his hand over his heart and smiled at me, saying, "Sympathetic strings; that's what we call us. Have you heard of sympathetic strings?"

I humbly replied, "No. What are they?"

"Like a violin," he explained, "there is a string that is the primary string, and when it is plucked, another string will respond and vibrate. They are sympathetic strings. You (a Christian) would say, 'I resonate with you,'" and as he opened his hands in a gesture of welcome, he assured me, "That is how *we* are."

In that particular moment in time and space, two devotees' souls vibrated: one for Krishna, and the other for Christ, both hearts singing for their God, sharing their love for the Lord and for other human beings. The beauty of our souls recognizing each other, and resonating with the love of God, outside of time and space, understanding each other in ways words cannot describe, filled my heart with awe and wonder. This has happened before in my life, each and every time creating awareness within me of divine presence, not only in a mystical sense but physically in this body, all senses fully engaged, the mind making connections of intuitive resonance and the heart connecting at the soul level with another human being, speaking a soul language I completely and intuitively understand. I recognize and become fully aware that I am at once alive, present, and eternal.

One time in seminary, when I first encountered a new student on campus, we discovered we were both meditators. At our first meditation, it was as if we had been soul friends from long before, perhaps meeting once again to awaken to deeper truths and clearer awareness of God. It happens like that sometimes. God opens us to awakening to higher consciousness at deeper levels, all at the right time. Another time in a restorative yoga teacher training, as I lay still in a pose, my heart *chakra* (I'll be discussing chakras in more depth in Chapter 7) released a blockage that I didn't know was there. The stuck energy released from my heart into the space around me, and I lay there, in awe of what God was doing in me, flowing new energy for greater healing and deeper awareness of the presence of God within me.

It is good to be alive. I feel only gratitude. Gratitude for all that is.

## ～ 3 ～

# The Inner Landscape –
# *The Crucial Pilgrimage*

> We will never fully know God until we
> come to know ourselves thoroughly.
>
> —*Julian of Norwich*[23]

## The Spirituality of Pilgrimage

The spiritual path is an inner pilgrimage. A pilgrimage is the universal practice of going to a sacred place to make offerings, ask favors, or share in the powers of a holy person, spirit, or deity.[24] Pilgrimage is also a form of intentional ritual that brings you in touch with the divine in a palpable way, opening up new inner experiences and revelations. An inner pilgrimage brings you in touch with the soul, the inner longing of the heart. Mary Oliver, in her poem "The Old Poets of China," expresses the soul's desire to go inward, to discover the depths of our own souls:

### The Old Poets of China[25]

Wherever I am, the world comes after me.
It offers me its busyness. It does not believe
that I do not want it. Now I understand
why the old poets of China went so far and high
into the mountains, then crept into the pale mist.

Embarking on a pilgrimage of travel opens the possibilities to discovering something about the world, a culture, a people, a religion, their spirituality, and perhaps most importantly, about yourself. My first pilgrimage was to the Navajo Nation in Arizona. Our mission team departed from Galveston, Texas, tools and Mardi Gras beads in tow to assist the church in teaching a vacation bible school to the children and to offer cleaning, organizing, and handiwork on the church buildings and grounds. At the time, I didn't realize how much I would receive from this pilgrimage until I began to experience the Navajo people. Their deep, abiding joy began to affect my soul.

A Navajo woman in her late 80s came to our dinner. Her long gray, black hair braided down her back was neat and reflected a woman who cared about her appearance. Her long flowing skirt and billowy blouse exuded her femininity, even with her age. She was exquisitely beautiful with dark eyes that reflected deep pools of living water; they shone with a depth of soul. She smiled at me. We didn't speak the same language, but our smiles connected our hearts.

Her translator asked if the older woman could touch me, and I said yes. She began to touch my arm, rubbing her hand along my skin, and I realized she wanted to "feel me." She smiled. Her translator told me that she loved my skin, and then asked me to touch her arm. Her skin was dry, yet I loved the deep, bronze color. I always wanted dark bronze skin. This wise woman told me, through the translator, that living out here had drained the moisture out of her skin, just as the government had drained the life out of her family. She was the youngest child of five in her family. They had lived on the land, keeping sheep. One day the US government came and took her family from her. All of the other children were taken to attend a school where they would learn to read and write. But she remained, the youngest, to take care of the sheep for the family. She was abandoned, separated from her kin, left behind as if she did not matter. But she had a resilient spirit.

As she told me her story, I saw the pain show through her eyes, and then the resignation, and then the acceptance. She was an old woman now, showing me through her dry skin that her tears had long since dried too. It was because of her that I vowed to never go on a vacation again that didn't involve some sort of ministry, or a pilgrimage, that would give me a glimpse into another's soul and into my own, stretching my perspective and giving me a greater understanding of the interconnectedness of all of God's people—and all of God's creation. This exchange between us on that fateful day, which still brings tears to my eyes, brought me closer to the heart of God, and to the beautiful child of God before me. We were both the same: two souls longing for human connection and love. Different skin, different life stories, yet both women and children of God.

My pilgrimages have since included holy lands of many faith traditions. It is wonderful to experience pilgrimage in a country whose culture, history, religion, and people have so much to teach me. My soul hungers for an authentic encounter of God in these places, among people different from me, even among people of different religions. The sacred is always sacred, if we have the eyes to see.

My soul also hungers for an authentic encounter with God interiorly, wherever I am—in my own home, my own body, my own heart. Even in the most ordinary of places, in the everyday, God can be found. I don't need to travel the world over searching for God, for God is always with me. I have known that ever since I was a little girl. God has been there in the silence, in the wind, in the trees, in nature, in my soul.

Our inner landscape is where we do our deep soul work. Out in the world with people our souls touch, we see mirrors of ourselves—ready to teach us within if we are willing to truly see the reflection looking back at us. When we pilgrimage into our inner landscape, this is where we find our souls and the spirit of God within us. The most sacred work we can ever do is our own inner work. This is the work that shapes our lives, our relationships, and ultimately our ability to serve others. This is where we come to terms with our childhood experiences and feelings, our disappointments, our regrets. This is where we make peace with our life, with ourselves.

There are so many ways to do our inner work. The practice of spiritual direction helps to get in touch with God's presence, listening for the presence and movement of God in life. In spiritual direction, as I guide another soul on their soul journey, I encourage prayer, journaling, the reading of Scripture and sacred writings, meditation, and sometimes a journey beyond the ordinary.

I still love to listen to God in the wind, and when I'm not in nature and want to go into my inner landscape, I find an hour, usually in the evening, to get on my mat and flow. My inner guide moves me in the direction that my body and spirit want and need to go. I am my own teacher. My body knows what I need. The Spirit of Christ stays with me as I flow to my own breath or the rhythmic music on my playlist. Carl Jung describes the fruit of listening to your heart: "Your vision will become clear when you look into your heart. Who looks outside, dreams. Who looks inside, awakens."

## The Meaning of Life

We reach a point in our spiritual journey where we begin to ask the existential question of any lifetime, and one that has been asked over the history of humankind: *Who am I?* The asking of this question marks the beginning of our deepest inner pilgrimage. We ask it in our teenage years when we are trying to fit in with our classmates, and then again as we approach young adulthood, in college, in our studies and skills training, and as we embark on our changing adult career or vocation. As we become accomplished in our goals and aspirations, and gain more material possessions, we ask the question to ensure we have the strength and stamina to persevere, and more importantly, to ensure that we are on the "right track." Later in life, as we begin to reflect on our purpose in life, the question has a greater significance related to making a difference beyond ourselves.

*Who am I?* In my thirties, my answer was "I am a business woman who is in charge of a multi-million dollar software installation! I must get up and get going!" No time to hit the snooze button and sleep another ten minutes! (And sadly, "Never mind that I am grieving, I've got a job to do and people are counting on me.")

For me, that simple yet profound question continued to gnaw at me no matter how successful (or not so successful) I was on any given project or goal. I began to sense that I didn't really have the correct and complete answer to that question if I only defined myself as a career woman, a businesswoman, or what all moms know to be true in the world of working parents. (I was simply "Cameron's mom" in many circles.) God began nudging me to pray. My prayer life changed from one-way asking of God for what I needed and wanted, to discourse, and then to silence. I came to a point where all I wanted to do was sit in silence and pray. Even at work, I would often race off during lunch to be alone with God. Anti-social? Introvert? Only God knew. But it really was good news—I was being changed from the inside out.

I wear many hats in terms of our culture and our society. If I described myself even ten years ago, my description would be different than today's. Today, I am an Episcopal priest serving a small and loving community in central southwest Houston in the Episcopal Diocese of Texas. I am a spiritual director. I am a Benedictine Oblate with the World Community for Christian Meditation. I am a meditator and yoga practitioner. I am a certified 200-hour Yoga Alliance and Nosara Yoga Educator, working on my additional 300-hour certification. I am a mystic and a contemplative. I am a wife, mother, mother-in-law, grandmother, daughter, sister, cousin, and servant of two independent-minded cats who share my home with me. My ecumenical and interfaith work brings me to reach out and build bridges in our communities with other churches and faith organizations. But aside from all the labels, categories, and identities, I simply am. I AM.

We all have "identities" by which we define ourselves. My list has changed over the years as my career and my passions have evolved, and it is growing shorter, by my own doing. I can honestly and gratefully say I have moved into the "second half of life" as Richard Rohr describes it. Sometimes my ego does win and drive me forward, but for the most part, I try and listen for God's still, small voice, the "sound of sheer silence," (1 Kings 19:12) to guide and lead me forward. My life is not yet completed, so my answer to "Who am I?" may shift again in the future. But for now, I know one thing for sure. I am a child of God and a bearer of the divine light of God. And so are you.

We are all searching for our purpose. We seek to know who we are and what we are supposed to do. Interestingly, Anodea Judith, author, psychologist, and teacher, brings this search closer to home, closer to the body. She says, "It is not the meaning of life we seek as much as it is our aliveness. Once we have our aliveness, the meaning of life becomes obvious. When you feel fully alive, you know what you're here for."[26] Feeling fully alive is freeing, liberating, and a participation in the energy flow of the divine. I want this feeling always.

Yoga is teaching me to more fully appreciate and engage with the process of feeling alive in my body, with my energy, with my breath, and with the world around me. Yoga practice has its physically observable benefits too, sculpting the body noticeably on the outside to reflect what is being sculpted within: strength, vitality, and a deeper congruence with the mind of Christ, the consciousness of God's presence everywhere and within everyone, including myself!

## A Path of Discovery: The Path of Meditation

When Christian meditation began taking me inward into my own heart, I began to hear God in ways I hadn't since I was a little girl. I remember when I was five years old how much I enjoyed sitting in our backyard and listening quietly to the wind moving through the trees, and saying to my girlfriend, "Shhhh...listen to the wind; listen, it's God." (Instinctively, even as a child, I knew the presence of *ruach*.) That same kind of listening is the listening of meditation, the listening within the deepest part of my heart. It is the pilgrimage from the head to the heart, moving us from intellect to experience, from thinking to feeling, from structure to creativity, from *doing* to *being*. This is the journey of aliveness that is so needed in our world today.

The practice of Christian meditation, the silent prayer of the heart, is a path to self-discovery. In Christian meditation, or contemplative prayer, we let go into the pure presence of God. We may repeat a mantra or sacred word silently, interiorly, as we rest in God's presence. The sacred word may fall away and we rest in a vast, quiet space momentarily, until the mind begins to think again, taking us back into thinking about the experience. And we start again with the mantra.

In Christian terms, the path of meditation is self-emptying, or *kenosis*, when we have no thoughts, words, or images and we simply rest in God's gaze, allowing God to speak to us in the silence. The letting go of the ego, the thinking and controlling mind, is the hardest part. Just as soon as I reach a peaceful place, the "monkey mind" starts working again, and I'm thinking that I'm sitting there, that I'm meditating, or I'm reviewing my to-do list and my hopes and dreams. I usually find myself dreaming about someone or some event that I am planning. My thoughts and my ego want to direct and control everything, even my relationship with God and myself. The goal is to let the ego fall away and allow God's Spirit within to speak.

Meditation is the spiritual practice of letting go of the ego and controlling the mind. We sit for twenty minutes or more, saying the mantra interiorly, which quiets the mind. It is a practice and not always successful. Just as athletes train their bodies, sitting in meditation trains the mind to be still and quiet. Training the mind to be calm, to relax into the present moment, and to rest with no thoughts brings peace. Meditation teaches us the gift of presence, and we can bring this peace and presence off the meditation mat or yoga mat and into our daily lives.

When I first began meditating, I was a type-A personality focused on achievement and multi-tasking. It was a survival technique for me to pull myself out of a life of boredom and intermittent mild depression. Accomplishing a busy to-do list and work projects gave me purpose. What was lacking was a full and complete spiritual connection to God for direction and purpose, and a holistic approach to life. All I knew was for my survival: I needed to stay busy, get things done, and do them well. That was my identity, and I am sure I was hard to live with. My husband wanted my big project to end, and he told me he wanted "me" back. I was driven, focused, and unwavering, at the expense of my friendships, my health, and our marriage.

Meditation slowed me down. Meditation helped me enter a "heart space" that otherwise was inaccessible. Meditation was the path to discovering the right-brain creative, feminine aspect of myself, an unknown part of that had been lost since childhood. The practice of meditation helped me to understand when I was in a mild depression and gave me the patience to sit with God as I prayed through it, asking for strength and the grace for it to lift, and then resting in God's presence to heal me. Meditation changed me, and it saved my life.

Research shows that meditation changes the brain by increasing the amount of gray matter in the insula and sensory regions, the auditory and sensory cortex. Important research by Dr. Sara Lazar, neuroscientist at Massachusetts General Hospital and Harvard Medical School, was published in the Washington Post, summarizing the results of her studies of the impact of meditation on the brain. Here's what she found:

> We found that long-term meditators have a thickening in four regions of the brain: the posterior cingulate, which is involved in mind wandering and self-relevance; the left hippocampus, which assists in learning, cognition, memory and emotional regulation; the temporo-parietal junction, associated with perspective-taking, empathy and compassion; and the brain stem area called the Pons, where regulatory neurotransmitters are produced. The amygdala, the fight or flight part of the brain that responds to anxiety, fear, and stress, actually got smaller. [27]

When you're mindful, you're paying attention to your breathing, to sounds, to the present moment experience, and shutting cognition down. It stands to reason that your senses would be enhanced.

The yogis have known this for millennia. Modern science is now catching up and affirming what they have known. For us today, it's all good news!

## The Lost Contemplative Tradition Emerges

In the modern Western world, our minds control our activities, what we think, and even what we feel. Many of us have lost touch with our feelings, our center, our groundedness in God. Directly offsetting this, however, is the rediscovery and renewal of meditation, which is rapidly changing the landscape of our souls and our communities.

Some say the shift toward meditation in the West was set in motion at the first World's Parliament of Religions in Chicago in 1893, when an encounter between the east and the west began a shift in consciousness on a global scale. The Asian ascetic, Vivekananda, introduced the Eastern philosophy of yoga into the conversation, changing the trajectory of consciousness from that point forward. The Parliament has been praised as the birth of the interfaith movement and as signaling the emergence of the comparative study of religion.[28]

The contemplative movement of Christian meditation in the West resurfaced in the mid-20th century from its disappearance during the Renaissance, with the teachings of Thomas Merton, Thomas Keating, John Main, Laurence Freeman, and many others. These teachers began to spread the gift of Christian meditative practices that are known as *the prayer of the heart*, which were drawn from the early Christian mystics (also referred to as centering prayer and contemplative prayer).

During seminary in 2006, we pondered if we were in the midst of another Great Awakening, such as the one that began on Azusa Street in Los Angeles, California in 1906. That awakening was characterized by ecstatic spiritual experiences, speaking in tongues, and was described as a Pentecost—even by modern standards. These days, the spiritually exploratory attitudes influencing our society—such as so many people in the US crossing denominational lines, religious traditions expanding their purview, and even Pope Francis' reshaping of many views and practices—are convincing indications that we are going through an awakening or an emergence that brings forth new forms of religious expression.

So, what *is* emerging? It seems to be a higher level of "consciousness": an increasing awareness of the divine presence within oneself and in all others, including all of creation, which is emerging among *all* traditions, at least to some extent.

Christianity as it has historically been taught and enacted in the Western Church is being called to change—to "mix it up," as the young people say. Many young people—in the United States and Europe in particular—are secularizing spirituality. We see this in their "I'm spiritual but not religious" perspective that calls for a heart-based renewal of religion and celebrates our very humanity and the gift of our planet Earth.

The contemplative movement, which in its essence integrates spirituality into everyday life, reminds us that we touch the soul of our humanity when we breathe, when we quiet our minds, sit in silence, and listen to that still, small voice of God within. "Be still and know that I am God" (Psalm 46:10). It is similar to the eastern practice of meditation, which is likewise one way that we find our souls again, regardless of what religious tradition we employ as we sit in silence and listen for divine guidance that speaks to our souls. Meditation, according to the yogic tradition, is a key component of the science of human experience, so we will explore it in more detail now.

## Into the Silence

The mind is an integral component of our very human-ness, and it likes to be in control. In meditation, we train the mind to slow down and be still, and we observe the subtle movement of our thoughts and the energy in our bodies and our hearts. Our bodies will teach us everything, if only we will listen to them. What are they telling us when we feel heat or cold, contraction or expansion, vibration or stillness, hardness or openness? What primary feeling is our heart expressing to us at this moment?

Meditation can strip away the external influences and bring us to a still state where we can notice, pay attention, and investigate. And then, while still in meditation, we can let go of even the noticing, and rest in the presence of God's universal healing power and love. Jesus spoke of the act of meditation in Matthew 6:6:

> "Whenever you pray, go into your room and shut the door and pray to your Father who is in secret; and your Father who sees in secret will reward you."

In the *Shambhala* tradition, as described by Chögyam Trungpa, the late Buddhist meditation master, meditation is a very basic act:

> "Sitting on the ground, assuming a good posture, and developing a sense of our spot, our place on this earth. This is the means of rediscovering ourselves in to genuine reality, without any expectations or preconceptions....It is about simply training our state of being so that our mind and body can be synchronized. Through the practice of meditation, we can learn to be without deception, to be fully genuine and alive."[29]

Meditation gets us in touch with the deepest part of our soul that we may find awareness of God within. When we find soul union with God, it is not merely a spiritual act that requires we ignore our bodies, as if our bodies no longer matter. They matter greatly, because our bodies will continue to be the temples that house our souls as long as we are alive. As St. Paul encouraged:

> "Or do you not know that your body is a temple of the Holy Spirit within you, which you have from God, and that you are not your own? For you were bought with a price; therefore glorify God in your body" (1 Corinthians 6:19-20).

Our bodies, as temples of God's Spirit within, help us to be fully alive, to live in this world, experiencing all that being alive has to offer: joys, sorrows, playfulness, work, prayer, rest. Meditation helps us to reconnect with our center again and to remember that inside of these amazing, miraculous bodies is a soul that can experience the vastness of the universe, the vastness of God. The practice of meditation helps us to touch that deep part of our soul and practicing it helps us to put all things in perspective.

The discovery of the inner Self, the true Self and God's purpose for us as we live into that knowledge, is a process of unfolding grace. When we take the view that it is a process, we can allow God the space to move in our lives in God's time, *kairos* time, rather than in our time. Whether we move in a hurried fashion or slowly, we can trust that God's time is unfolding in our lives exactly at the right time.

When we are standing in the darkness holding a lantern, the light of the lantern creates a circle around us, so that we can see enough for a few steps in front of us. If there were no darkness and everything was always brightly illuminated, we could see completely where God is leading us, and this might be frightening for us, leading us far from our comfort zone. God shows us only the next step or two, so that we are willing to step forward as God leads us on the way. This process of self-discovery into our own calling is as gentle as we need it to be. We only have to be willing to take the next step forward. It's a journey, a pilgrimage into our own true and sacred nature.

When we meditate, we can have a sacramental moment, coming to know the truth of the divine light of our spirit within us meeting God's Spirit, if only for a moment. And even more, a meditation practice brings us into the process of ongoing conversion, in which, as Laurence Freeman, Order of St. Benedict (OSB), priest, monk, and leader of the World Community for Christian Meditation says in his book, *Light Within: Inner Path of Meditation*:

"We arrive at a mindfulness of the one Christ present in our hearts and in the world, not remembering Jesus by turning our imagination to the past...but mindful of his presence in the present moment....We awaken to this presence at the deepest level of consciousness."[30]

In the depths of silence, meditation is a pilgrimage on the path of awakening to higher consciousness, to Christ deep within.

## Inner Beauty

The benefits of yoga go much deeper than outer beauty. The greatest benefits go deep into the landscape of your body, which has many layers, each of which yoga touches, shifts, and heals. The muscular body is strengthened and moves with greater ease. The skeletal body is realigned for less stress on the joints. The energy body gets reset for clarity and ease. The mind becomes still and less chaotic and less distracted. The soul may rest easily and be at peace.

Yoga *asanas* or physical postures are healing and therapeutic. The practice of yoga poses takes us on a pilgrimage within each time we get on our mats. Experiencing the movements brings awareness to sensations, breath, and the ease or discomfort of the poses. Experiencing the breath brings the present moment rushing in. Practicing yoga *asanas* and flow brings challenges and emotions to the surface, sometimes quite unexpectedly. On more than one occasion, as I lay folded over one leg in pigeon pose, with the largest muscle in my body experiencing a deep stretch, spontaneous tears begin to flow, followed by deep sobs, and then a release comes from a place deep within. I didn't even know I was holding something painful that needed letting go: sadness, a regret, heartache, anger, or frustration—but my body knew.

Discovering held emotions through their release from the body is an aspect on the journey of self-healing, a pilgrimage of inner healing.

The experience of YogaMass, which engages body, mind, soul, and spirit, is a spiritual pilgrimage of beauty in the presence of community. It is a process of discovering that God is in the midst of all of us gathered; as we discover the presence of God within, we discover that God's divine spark is within each other as well. We discover that we are no different than the person next to us, as each of us is simply trying to do the best we can. God is present within each of us, but we are not all aware of this, and if we are, we are not *always* aware; we forget.

The gift of YogaMass is to bring that awareness into a communal gathering, a community ritual, so that we bring the reality of God into conscious awareness once again. God is always present in our consciousness; we simply aren't always aware of God's presence—and sometimes we reject God altogether, desiring instead what our ego grasps for at that moment. In YogaMass, as we become more and more consciously aware of God: we are bridging the divide between our own minds and the consciousness of God.

We consciously participate with our body as our temple. Our body is our "earthen vessel" or clay jar that allows our spiritual treasure to reach its fullest spiritual potential. St. Paul teaches, "But we have this treasure in jars of clay, to show that the surpassing power belongs to God and not to us" (2 Corinthians 4:7). It is our responsibility to care for our earthen vessels, our clay jars, and to nourish them well during our lifetime. But the real treasure is the seat of the soul, the heart and the spirit, integrated deeply within our bodies. The heart and the spirit are what we seek in our inner journey, for them, as our essence, to be in communion with God.

## The Pilgrimage of Gratitude

Our reconnection with the soul and re-discovery of communion with God within is the awakening that brings us into the gift of the present "now," teaching us what we are to learn in this moment, in this phase of life. A friend told me it began for her when she was in a bad car accident that found her convertible rolling and rolling and landing on an embankment. Her life was spared. Her soul saw something it had not seen before. She awakened to the soul within, and to her body that had so graciously housed her soul all these years. She vowed: no more abuse, only care. No time to waste, it is now all gift, pure gift. This new chapter, new beginning of her life was now presenting itself like a wake-up call from the universe. Get busy—get going! Life is precious: a reminder of the gift of life. Tend to yourself.

I had a similar life experience over twenty years ago that changed my perspective on how I see myself, others, and God. It was life changing: the death of my first husband by suicide. The precious gift of life and the impermanence of it all stared me in the face, and I could not hide. I had two choices: to drown in my sorrows and become angry and bitter, or to begin the difficult and arduous process of deep inner exploration and healing. I had to forgive him, and myself, for my own participation in his feelings of desperation. I had to look in the mirror deeply to search my soul for darkness and light, ugliness and beauty, pain and liberation. They were all there, real and present. Slowly, and over time, I began to find the deepest awareness of the sanctity of it all—God's presence even in the suffering, and in the lessons to be learned. Life clearly was giving me no shortcuts.

None of us want to experience such a tragedy, and yet when such tragedy happens, we can grow into a sense of gratefulness for another chance, an opportunity to learn and grow, and the opportunity to see God face to face. We can be grateful for what each event teaches us. In our stubbornness and "sleepiness," sometimes it takes a loud knock on our door to wake us up to the path to wholeness that has been there all along, waiting for us to step onto it and begin the journey of the heart, the journey home to God.

A heart of gratitude propels us forward on the spiritual path to a greater wholeness. The journey to wholeness, with gratitude for what is, even as challenging as it all may be, is one of the greatest gifts of being alive, as deeper and deeper healing unfolds. On this journey, it is imperative to attend to the soul and the spirit in a holistic way, with the awareness of body, mind, soul, and spirit as inseparable and integral to the path of healing and wholeness. To live in the fullness of God, there is no time like the present, and truly that is all there really is: this present moment and its eternal essence.

The poet Rumi illumines the path of inner pilgrimage with its timeless quality:

### Forget Your Life

Forget your life.
Say *God is Great.* Get up.
You think you know
what time it is.
It's time to pray.

You've carved so many little figurines, too many.
Don't knock on any random door like a beggar.
Reach your long hand out
to another door, beyond where
you go on the street, the street
where everyone says, "How are you?"
and no one says How aren't you?

Tomorrow you'll see what you've broken and torn tonight,
thrashing in the dark. Inside you
there's an artist
you don't know about.
He's not interested in how things
look different in moonlight.

If you are here unfaithfully with us,
you're causing terrible damage.
If you've opened your loving to God's love,
you're helping people you don't know
and have never seen.

Is what I say true?
Say yes quickly,
if you know, if you've known it
from before the beginning of the universe.[31]

The pilgrimage to the Spirit of God is the greatest pilgrimage
of all. When we look deep within, what we find there vastly
changes everything.

## ～4～

# Self-Discovery –
# *Finding the True Self*

The ultimate abandonment of one's role is not to have a self
as a fixed point of reference; it is the freedom to manifest God
through one's own uniqueness...For Christians, it is to be a kind
of Fifth Gospel: to become the word of God and to manifest
God rather than the false self, with its emotional programs
for happiness and attachments to various roles, including the
most spiritual. When you have been liberated from them all,
you are in a space that is both empty of self and full of God.

*–Thomas Keating*[32]

## Treasure

In the last chapter, we discussed the importance of inner and
outer pilgrimage. In this chapter, we will explore the discoveries
we make during the inner pilgrimage. *To know oneself is to discover
a treasure.* Treasures are things of great value that we long for, often
hidden or kept in a safe place. For some, treasures are people;
for others they are things. For some, the greatest treasure is God
"out there," and for others, the golden treasure is God "within."
It doesn't have to be an either/or, but one without the others
creates imbalance.

We might ask ourselves: "What do I value most? Are my
treasures people, things, God, or myself? Which are temporal and
passing, and which are permanent and eternal?"

You've heard it said about money (perhaps Americans' most valued treasure) that, "You can't take it with you." It seems apparent that most Americans value money over anything else. Except, perhaps football. The nearby football stadium packs over 90,000 people on a Sunday, while our little church struggles to fill the pews. Our culture drives our values and thus what we treasure most. I wonder: don't we as a society value our spiritual nature? Do we value a spiritual path? Why has God—or worshipping God—become less important in our collective lives?

I feel happy when I hear people say they value their families most. Families are where we all hope to find the greatest love, acceptance, and belonging. Families are hopefully where we learn that *we* are of great value. I wonder how many people really feel that they are a treasure? What are the messages we received in our early years? What are the messages we receive from our self-talk now?

It is in discovering our self-worth that we discover our pot of gold, and it is *inner gold*, as Robert Johnson, the great Jungian analyst termed it. The spiritual path is the path to recognizing that truth, our inner gold. Do we ever consider that the pot of gold we are looking for is here all along: God everywhere, and God within?

Our God, as best as we are able to understand and use language to describe a mystery, is both transcendent and immanent. A transcendent God is a God who is out there in the vast universe, transcending space and time, the God who created all. A theology of immanence describes God as indwelling, inherent, of remaining within. If God indwells in the universe, in time, and in all of creation, then God dwells in us too. Jesus the Christ was the perfect manifestation of the indwelling of God, Word made Flesh. The spiritual path for the rest of us is the path to awakening to the indwelling of God within us, discovering our inherent divinity within these human bodies.

Jesus says, "The kingdom of God is within you." When I close my Eucharist services at Grace with the Blessing over the people, I like to say these words, "And may God the Father, the Son, and the Holy Spirit, be among you and *within* you, this day and always." It is important to me to acknowledge God's presence within and share it as a spiritual teaching. I hope the people hear these words with the ears of their hearts.

Many people ask me, "But how do I get to the place where I know this? I've been told it, but I want to *believe* it." Another perspective I hear is, "I cannot believe this. I am not God, so it can't be true that God is present within me, that I am divine. Only Jesus is God." My answer is always that Jesus wished us to know this truth:

> "In a little while the world will no longer see me, but you will see me; because I live, you also will live. On that day you will know that I am in my Father, and you in me, and I in you" (John 14:19-20).

The spiritual journey is to make this discovery that God is within you. No one can do it for you, although it does take others to help you begin the journey, and to resume the journey when you have stepped off the path or taken a detour. Therapy has been for me a part of this self-discovery journey. I cannot separate the process of therapy from my spiritual journey because they are like a tapestry, each thread of realization is woven in with others: my life experiences, my stories, my feelings, and my experience of God. I preach that therapy is one of the greatest gifts you can give yourself. It is not something to be ashamed of; it is an essential part of our work of self-discovery. It is integral to understanding your behaviors, your emotions, and your belief system, and it is a component of the path to self-knowledge and emotional, psychological, and spiritual maturity. Therapy, along with forgiveness and other psychological and emotional healing modalities such as tapping for thought freedom (TFT) and emotional freedom (EFT), yoga, and meditation, aids in bringing you to the path of individuation, to knowing who you are and what you believe, not what someone else told you to believe. And we each have to walk this road ourselves.

Jesus taught that self-discovery—which brings new life—is available to us all when he said,

> "Ask, and you will receive. Search, and you will find. Knock, and the door will be opened to you. For everyone who asks, receives. Whoever seeks, finds. And to everyone who knocks, the door is opened" (Matthew 7:7-8, Common English Bible).

There is so much to unpack in this teaching, but for now, let's begin with the key words—the verbs, "ask and search." Some translations use "seek" for "search," but the word "search" is more powerful. Seek is to search for, to try to find, to ask for something or someone. Search means to *carefully* look for someone or something that often may be hidden. This is what Jesus describes in this story that teaches a spiritual lesson:

> "The kingdom of heaven is like treasure hidden in a field, which someone found and hid; then in his joy he goes and sells all that he has and buys that field" (Matthew 13:44).

What we treasure, what we value most and hold as special and important to us drives how we behave, what we do, and how we spend our time, energy, and resources. The depth of our desire drives the depth of our search. In spiritual direction, I try to help people see what they are valuing by asking questions such as, "How is your prayer life? Are you spending time with God?"

Jesus identifies the kingdom of Heaven as a treasure, one so valuable that the one who finds it would sell everything she has to obtain it. That's an all-or-nothing kind of response, the kind of response we often have when we fall in love: "I want to spend the rest of my life with this person." Or, "I'll go anywhere with you, as long as I am with you." And, "Till death do us part." That person has become our lifelong treasure, the one we have been searching for to share our journey with us. As a human being, we want that kind of connection and companionship. We are hardwired for connection. It is the instinctual basis for how our species continues. Socially, we desire to have friends with whom we can share our joys, heartaches, and struggles. We desire the deep soul intimacy of a soul mate. We long for intimate connection and will do almost anything for it.

## The Spirituality of Searching and Finding the Self

My heart is grateful for my teachers, friends, mentors, and soul mates along my journey, whose presence in my life, willingness to listen as I wrestle, and guidance to deeper discoveries have enriched my life and assisted me in the process of spiritual awakening to a greater consciousness. A trusted friend and guide is The Very Reverend Pittman J. McGehee, Episcopal priest and Jungian analyst. He helped me understand the spiritual path as liberating and freeing, not confining and rule-based. Pittman defines spirituality in this way:

> "To transfer the transcendent into the immanent through experience and reflection."

Spiritual practices help us to make this transfer, this journey along the continuum of "God out there" to "God in here." Every spiritual practice we engage in can provide an opening for the discovery of the immanent God. You may try some and find they don't fit. Other practices may work better for you; keep those. I am a meditator, and it is the door for me to enter into the most profound relationships with God, my Self, and other beautiful souls. But it isn't for everyone, and that's okay. I encourage you to find what works for you and stick with it. If it stops feeding your soul, find another practice! That's what a journey is all about.

The journey of self-discovery includes getting in touch with the deep-seated emotional memories that we carry with us. I am deeply grateful to my nutritionist, acupuncturist, spiritual friends, tai chi instructors, and yoga teachers for helping me understand the depths of the human body to retain memories and emotions. You may have heard the saying: "We have issues in our tissues." Yoga helps in the practice of letting go of these emotions that we carry within our bodies, not just the emotions themselves but also the effects of the emotions that we carry in our bodies long after the cause or experience has passed.

McGehee reminds me that our body and soul are interconnected and inseparable. In everyday language we say things like, "You broke my heart," and "It made me sick to my stomach." We experience our emotions *in these bodies*. We experience life with our hearts and our feelings, so deeply that we carry our emotions at the cellular level, sometimes for a lifetime. Yogis have known this for thousands of years. I place my hands in prayer over my heart with the deepest gratitude that the science of yoga has made its way to the West.

Ida Rolf, founder of Structural Integration and the Rolfing technique, understands the body to consist of energy:

> "A human being is basically an energy field operating in the greater energy field of the earth; particularly significant is that energy known as the gravitational field."[33]

Ida Rolf also said, "The body is the psyche in three dimensions." The dimensions are inseparable, not body *and* soul but body/soul. I have decided to use the term Body/Soul to describe the non-duality of our being-ness. We are not both body and soul, we are an integrated body/soul, and we are also an integrated body, mind, soul, and spirit. The Taoist tradition speaks to the connection of body and soul with spiritual realization:

> Taoist alchemy assumes the primacy of the physical body in the process of self-realization. The psychological and cosmic forces of the trigrams of the I Ching are stored in the internal organs of the body and are the basic material for the experience of Tao....The Chinese notion of Tao coincides with Jung's postulation of the *unus mundus*, the unity of existence which underlies the duality of psyche and matter, the psycho-physical background of existence. In this light, in the world of inner experience, East and West follow similar paths symbolically.[34]

I practice self-reflection on my mat with the perspective of unity of all that exists. It is the ongoing work of understanding myself and all that is around me. As my teacher Robert Boustany instructs me on how the bones, muscles, connective tissue, and energy channels work within my body, I have a deeper appreciation for the miracle that I am, that we all are. Going deeper into Yogic meditation, discovering the presence of energy and energy channels opens me to the possibilities within the unseen realms. Going deeper in *Savasana* and meditation, the body melts away and disappears, leaving the subtle body to flow into the vastness of the universe. For Christians, this is the vastness of God's all-knowing omnipresence in all of creation, this vastness of which we are all a part.

Just as yoga is a spiritual practice, and worship is an act of spiritual devotion to the Creator, Redeemer, and Sustainer God, the blend of yoga and worship together as YogaMass is a spiritual practice. Participating in YogaMass makes space for you to search for and touch the immanent God within to discover and find the beauty of God's vast creation within. YogaMass allows for an experience of being human: body, mind, soul, and spirit in forward folds, heart openers, and side stretches for experiencing life-force energy moving within you. YogaMass is an experience that the church can offer on the journey of self-discovery, celebrating the spiritual experience of *being alive* in our human bodies.

## Discovery Changes Us from the Inside Out

When we have a moment of discovery, the world opens up for us in a way that we couldn't see or imagine before. Everything becomes new. We feel alive! This happened to me at age 10, when I was in the fourth grade. Optometrist assistants came to my elementary school every six months to perform eye exams on students. My eye exam indicated that I needed to visit an eye doctor. I don't remember much about the visit, except that I felt embarrassed, like I was lacking in some way. Those old feelings of imperfection—even at such a young age—swirled through me. After being fitted for my new glasses, my mother drove me home. The first thing I did was what I always did: I went outside to be alone in nature. I remember sitting on the front porch looking up at the large oak tree in our front yard. I was totally amazed at the leaves on that tree. I could see each individual green leaf, as I had never seen them before, and I could see them gently moving and swaying with the wind. I took my glasses off and looked up, and realized this is what I had been seeing, a blur of green color without definition. I put my glasses back on and everything was crisp and bold. I was changed. I remember feeling so grateful, and yet so sad that I had been seeing less than what was possible, and yet not even knowing. We really don't know what we don't know.

I have always felt such gratitude for the people in my life who have led me forward, helping me to see clearly what is possible, to see what I might not have been able to see on my own. We imagine, we dream, we create, and then God leads us in a direction that is even beyond what we ever imagined or dreamed.

Jesus looked at them and said, "For mortals it is impossible, but for God all things are possible" (Matthew 19:26). The process of discovery ultimately belongs to each of us individually, and how remarkable and beautiful it is to discover along the way someone who guides us forward. We need each other. In community, with friends and soul mates, we learn to become more fully human. We learn about ourselves when we are in relationship with another. Sometimes we learn things about ourselves that we would rather not see, giving us the opportunity to learn and grow and change. We also learn about our own ability to love, to experience "*agape*," the love of charity, giving, and sharing with another human being because we see in them an image of God.

This kind of love reminds me of the Sanskrit greeting, *Namaste*, which means "The divine in me bows to the divine in you." Yoga practices usually end with the *Namaste* bow. Holding hands in prayer over the heart, and speaking the word *Namaste* with a deep bow, an outward and visible sign of acknowledging the presence of God within you and within me, is a gesture of *agape* love. It is like the Christian greeting of peace during a worship service where the Priest says, "Peace be with you," and the people respond, "And also with you." The gathered community then shares the peace with each other with handshakes or hugs. This time is set apart for us to share peace with each other, a love fest full of happiness and gratitude as we greet each other with smiles, hugs, and pure joy to be with each other once again. Peace, peace, peace. Namaste. The heart is happy.

## Giving Birth to That Which is Within You

I was invited to give a presentation to the Foundation for Contemporary Theology (FCT) in Houston. Over its nearly 30 year history, this foundation has brought religious scholars and thinkers to Houston for critical discussion and debate over theological issues that have informed American Christianity for more than two centuries. Speakers with religious perspectives on contemporary issues have sparked important conversation among people of all faiths, and those of no faith, seeking to find commonality as human beings with greater understanding of our differences. An FCT board member, Stuart Nelson (also our YogaMass sitar player), invited me to speak at their luncheon in my role as creator of YogaMass, a creative expression of faith outside of traditional worship experiences. It was also a designated week for the City of Houston called "Compassionate Houston Week," bringing people of all faith communities to serve together on compassion projects, attend lectures, and participate in discussions to foster a stronger community and a more compassionate city.

I took the occasion to dive more deeply into two of the Scriptures that I use in the YogaMass liturgy. These scriptures may be unknown to most Christians but they are a treasure—once hidden and now found. They are from the *Gospel of Thomas*, one of the early gospels discovered in northern Egypt only recently, in 1945, that didn't make the canons for our New Testament Bible. Until the 20th century, Christians believed there were only four gospels: the gospels of Matthew, Mark, Luke and John. These were the gospels selected in the middle of the 4th century AD, after much prayer, discernment, and debate, for the canon of New Testament: the approved, authoritative Holy Scripture. The four Gospels of the New Testament proclaim the good news of Jesus by telling stories about his life and death—including his birth, ministry, miracles, teaching, last days, crucifixion, and resurrection. Additional books were selected to develop the sacred, authorized canon, 27 books in all; these include the Acts of the Apostles, letters written by Christian leaders to various communities and individuals, and the Book of Revelation.

I have discovered that many people today no longer ascribe to an external authoritative set of beliefs but rather to their own process of seeking, searching, and discovering their own experience that leads to faith in God. The *Gospel of Thomas* speaks to our post-modern age: *to those looking for spirituality and not "right belief."* In reviewing these texts with study groups, it is helpful to ponder why they may not have been selected as authorized canon—perhaps they were considered to be of secret knowledge, or of an esoteric wisdom tradition, or simply the loser of a struggle for "correct belief." Every student must discern for himself or herself what these other gospels may mean for them. Orthodoxy, or "right belief," is simply no longer accepted as the only path, especially by many Christians (and others) who prefer a spirituality of *Orthopraxy*, or "right practice." *Orthopraxy* focuses on the practice of following Jesus, while Orthodoxy is based on believing, using a soteriological perspective, one that is savior-oriented, believing that Jesus came to save us by dying for our sins.

Christianity has different emphases in the East and the West, and both have relevance for us today. Cynthia Bourgeault, Episcopal priest, author and wisdom school teacher examines the spirituality of the Christianity of the East, describing it as a sophiological Christianity. A sophiological Christianity focuses on the path of Jesus, and Bourgeault describes it as "emphasizing how Jesus is like us, how what he did in himself is something we are all also called to do in ourselves. By contrast, soteriology (Christianity from the West) tends to emphasize how Jesus is different from us—'begotten, not made,' belonging to a higher order of being, and hence uniquely positioned as our mediator."[35]

I wonder: Can we have a Christianity that is both soteriological *and* sophiological? From the sophiological perspective, it is the path of Jesus that brings the soul to a state of consciousness that is awakened to God's presence everywhere, all the time. This state of consciousness—this way of being—is described in one of the sayings in the *Gospel of Thomas*: Logion 51. I placed this teaching at the beginning of the Eucharistic prayer for YogaMass as a reminder that what we desire, we already have:

> "Yeshua replied, 'What you are looking for is already here. You simply have not recognized it'" (Logion 51).

Friends, what we are looking for is already here! As we hear these words, we are challenged to awaken to this truth and to help others awaken to this truth also. Or more rightly we are empowered to awaken to this truth: *God's light is in all of us*. The call for compassion and self-compassion run through this Gospel as we are called to wake up to what is within, to walk the path, and to grow into one's own full embodiment of God's divine light. This is a call to *embodied spirituality* as a path to self-discovery and then to full manifestation—and being present in one's body and in the present moment rather than living in the past or in the future.

The theologian Clement of Alexandria said, "To know oneself is to know God." Pittman McGehee stated these profound words at a conference: "My work is to become Pittman. That is all of our work, to become truly who we are."

The most compassionate and spiritual thing we can do for ourselves and others is to discover what is deep within each of us—our true basic goodness, the divine inner light in each of us shining brilliantly like a diamond or pure gold—and learn to live always in this awareness. If we are able to do that, we elevate our consciousness, and through the ripple effect, elevate the consciousness of humanity as well. Our churches can help us do this if the inner kingdom is allowed to resurface, to take its rightful place in the spiritual life, and to be nurtured through spiritual practice and corporate worship.

At the FCT luncheon, one attendee asked, "How do you find out who you really are?" Self-exploration is a journey to understand your personality, your psyche, your subconscious, and your body. The call is to understand all that self-exploration entails, and yet to go even deeper—into the very core and ground of your being, which is from God and of God and is God. Self-discovery ultimately leads to discovery of the Christ within, the Christ Consciousness. We too, like Jesus, are an incarnation, an embodied human being with a body, mind, soul and spirit, yearning for union with the Spirit of God. The Christian mystics knew this, and they wrote beautiful treatises from their deep inner knowing that we treasure.

Another attendee asked, "How do I discover who I am apart from who my culture, my family, my religious tradition tells me to be?" A dear, deceased friend and spiritual guide lived by this motto: "To remember who you really are, you have to forget who they told you to be." That remembering requires working toward self-individuation, standing in your truth, and always that you go back to spiritual practices, for they teach you to listen with the ear of the heart, to *your* heart. Listening to God in the silence of your heart teaches you everything you need to know.

## Uncovered Treasures for Our Time

The recent discoveries in the caves of the Dead Sea Scrolls at Qumran between the years 1947 and 1956 and the scriptures at Nag Hammadi in Upper Egypt in 1945 changed the landscape of the conversation of authority. We now understand more clearly that there were many and varied early Christian communities following the teachings of Jesus through the lens of a particular disciple. These teachings were as varied as the disciple who taught them (who was not necessarily the one who wrote them down), based on that disciple's fundamental beliefs and particular relationship with Jesus or views on his teachings, shared with the community he or *she* was leading or serving. The communities of Matthew, Mark, Luke and John were not the only Christian communities that flourished in the years after Jesus lived.

With these new discoveries near the Dead Sea and in Egypt, a whole new world has opened to scholars and many Christians that sheds light on the teachings of Jesus through these other Christian communities. Many Old Testament books, such as the Psalms, were also discovered in these findings, along with the four gospels that we inherited. And yet, there were more: the *Gospel of Thomas*, the *Gospel of Mary*, and the *Gospel of Philip* were among those found at Nag Hammadi. These findings have changed our understanding of early Christian communities—for those who have been open to studying them for new perspectives on the life, ministry, teachings, death, and resurrection of Jesus. Some question the validity of these newly resurfaced "non-canonical" gospels, claiming that they were gnostic in origin, and therefore not considered a credible source. This requires that we explore the meaning of the word gnostic.

"Gnostic" is a Greek word deriving from the root *gnosis*. Gnosis simply means knowledge. Many of the Nag Hammadi gospels have been labeled "Gnostic Gospels." The term "Gnostics" was given to those early Christian communities as a label to describe teachings deriving from "secret knowledge." The negative connotation wrapped around "secret" knowledge implied that these gospels were not legitimate because Jesus wouldn't have imparted certain knowledge or teachings to only a select few. I have often wondered why Native American spiritual practices, or yoga and meditation knowledge or techniques (just as examples), that were similarly passed down from spiritual leader or guru to student through oral tradition were not given the same negative connotation. What sociologically made one group "bad" while other groups were simply ignored? To that point, Cynthia Bourgeault reminds her readers that the scholar and author Karen King, has "come to recognize that Gnosticism is the inevitable shadow cast by the master story itself."[36] The late Walter Wink, theologian and scholar, also expressed that same conclusion in his work on human existence in his book, *Unmasking the Powers*:

> "One of the best ways to discern the weakness of a social system is to discover what it excludes from conversation...Because Gnosticism attempted, often in bizarre forms, to face sex and the inner shadow, it was declared heretical and driven underground, where it ironically became symbolic of the very repressed contents that it had attempted to lift up into the light. Gnosticism became Christianity's shadow."[37]

By understanding that a shadow in nature is created when an object obscures a light source from a particular location, we can see that the master story may certainly have obscured some good news revealed in the gospels uncovered and brought into the light only as recently as the late 19th and 20th centuries. I believe these Nag Hammadi gospels have more to teach us about who Jesus was, in light of healing and wholeness, at psychological and spiritual levels. Karen King says of the master story:

> According to the master story of Christian origins, Jesus passed down the true teaching to his male disciples during his lifetime...and, according to the master story, the full doctrine of Christianity was fixed by Jesus and passed on in the doctrines of the church. The *Gospel of Mary* instead suggests that the story of the gospel is unfinished. Christian doctrine and practice are not fixed dogmas that

one can only accept or reject; rather Christians are required to step into the story and work together to shape the meaning of the gospel in their own time.[38]

I wonder if the movement of people affirming their own spirituality apart from their inherited religious tradition is one aspect of the story continuing in our present time. The "Fifth Gospel," as Thomas Keating, Cistercian monk, author, and one of the founders of the Centering Prayer Movement, refers to this inner searching for truth in the opening quote of this chapter, is "embracing the freedom to manifest God—to become the word of God—through one's unique self," the self that has discovered the depths of God and one's own inner gold. The timing of discovering the ancient, non-canonical gospels is perfect, particularly during a time when individual and collective consciousness seems to be moving toward higher levels of understanding. These newly discovered gospels may be giving us a view of Jesus' teachings that clearly instructs us to engage this self-exploration.

The *Gospel of Thomas*, a treasure find, is a collection of sayings or teachings attributed to Jesus. Unearthed in Egypt in the middle of the last century, we are just beginning to understand its importance and impact. To provide a brief background: the text of the *Gospel of Thomas* exists in its entirety only in the Coptic version (the Egyptian language using Greek alphabet). Greek fragments of the Gospel were first found among the Oxyrhynchus papyri and published in 1897 and 1904. While the Coptic version dates to the early fourth century, some scholars estimate that the original text may have been composed late in the first century C.E., circa 80 AD or earlier, probably in Syria. Some scholars now believe the original version may have pre-dated the canonical gospels, and some speculate that the *Gospel of Thomas* may be the primitive "sayings" source for the synoptic Gospels Matthew, Mark and Luke.

Lynn C. Bauman describes the *Gospel of Thomas*, the *Gospel of Mary Magdalene* and the *Gospel of Philip* as "the Luminous Gospels, because they have a brilliance that illuminates a hidden aspect [an obscured light source] of the early Christian faith—the Jewish, Semitic and Oriental streams of the tradition." Bauman argues that "like all Semitic texts, the use of images and metaphors are highly favored over-against a more linear, propositional composition,"[39] providing a contrast between the metaphorical teaching (as reflected in these newly discovered gospels and in the canonical Gospel parables) and a story-like narrative (as reflected in the canonical *Gospels of Matthew, Mark, Luke, John,* and *The Acts of the Apostles)*.

For Bauman, these discoveries of *The Gospels of Thomas, Mary,* and *Philip* provide us now with a form of traditional wisdom (in the form of sayings or teachings) that also characterize the core of Jesus' wisdom teaching...(giving us) now, in an interesting way, two canons of texts: a Western and an Eastern canon. For Bauman, the "significance is that the needs of the two communities reflected an *alternative yet original version* of the wisdom and spiritual teachings coming from Jesus."[40] Throughout this book I will use Bauman's term "Eastern Canon" to describe these non-canonical gospels found at Nag Hammadi and to give them recognition as the gift they are for a more complete story of Jesus and his gift of salvation to the world.

The *Gospel of Thomas* is a wisdom text, a collection of 114 sayings or Logions in which Jesus instructs his followers in the process of transformation. *Thomas* is not alone in this type of Scripture; we also have a "long tradition of wisdom texts that includes Proverbs, Ecclesiastes, the Wisdom of Solomon, Pirke Aboth ('Sayings of the Fathers' included in the Mishnah), and the later collections of sayings of the Christian desert fathers"[41] and mothers in the 4th century, from which our monastic tradition emerged.

These wisdom teachings of Jesus in the *Gospel of Thomas*, where Jesus is called Yeshua, often sound strange, and yet, interestingly, many run parallel to our canonical gospels. For example, this passage is from the *Gospel of Thomas*:

> "His students said to him, 'Tell us about this kingdom of heaven of yours in heaven. What is it like?' Yeshua answered them. 'Let me compare it to a mustard seed, the smallest of all seeds. When it falls into prepared ground, it grows into a great tree capable of sheltering the birds of the sky'" (Logion 20).

Compare this to the *Gospel of Luke*:

> "He said therefore, 'What is the kingdom of God like? And to what should I compare it? It is like a mustard seed that someone took and sowed in the garden; it grew and became a tree, and the birds of the air made nests in its branches'" (Luke 13:18-19).

Another saying in the *Gospel of Thomas,* Logion 36, rings familiar:

> "Do not spend your time from one day to the next worrying about your outer appearance, what you wear and what you look like."

Here is the gospel given to us in the *Gospel of Matthew*:

> "Therefore I tell you, do not worry about your life, what you will eat or what you will drink, or about your body, what you will wear. Is not life more than food, and the body more than clothing?" (Matthew 6:25).

The *Gospel of Thomas* seems to be a gospel that teaches spiritual practices in ways not clearly made explicit in the canonical gospels. According to Cynthia Bourgeault, the Wisdom Jesus in the *Gospel of Thomas* brings forth "such perennial topics as mindfulness, presence, awakening, attention, vigilance, and non-possessiveness."[42] These are clearly attitudes of the heart that arise out of a contemplative spirituality. These are clearly topics for one seeking an intentional spiritual path of self-discovery and awakening to the presence of God. Just as clearly, they are topics that we can discuss with like-minded yoga and meditation practitioners who engage with contemplative spiritual practices, even across various religious traditions.

From the Jesus of the *Gospel of Thomas*, we are empowered to discover within. The Jesus of the *Gospel of Thomas* invites his followers to a path of inner seeing. Harold Bloom, in his Afterword to Marvin W. Meyer's translation of the *Gospel of Thomas*, describes Jesus as a teacher more than a savior:

> The Jesus of the Gospel of Thomas calls us to knowledge and not to belief, for faith need not lead to wisdom; and this Jesus is a wisdom teacher, gnomic and wandering, rather than a proclaimer of finalities....Nothing mediates the self for the Jesus of the Gospel of Thomas. Everything we seek is already in our presence, and not outside of our self. What is most remarkable in these sayings is the repeated insistence that everything is already open to you. You need but knock and enter. What is best and oldest in you will respond fully to what you allow yourself to see.[43]

In the canonical Gospels, Jesus repeatedly calls his followers to a new way of seeing:

And he said, 'Let anyone with ears to hear listen!'
(Mark 4:9)

The reason I speak to them in parables is that
'seeing they do not perceive, and hearing they do
not listen, nor do they understand.' With them
indeed is fulfilled the prophecy of Isaiah that says:
'You will indeed listen, but never understand, and
you will indeed look, but never perceive. For this
people's heart has grown dull, and their ears are
hard of hearing, and they have shut their eyes;
so that they might not look with their eyes, and
listen with their ears, and understand with their
heart and turn—and I would heal them.' But
blessed are your eyes, for they see, and your ears,
for they hear. (Matthew 13:13-16)

What deeper teaching is Jesus calling his disciples to see, hear,
understand, and embody? The more I study the non-canonical
"Eastern Canon" texts and their meanings from a contemplative
viewpoint, with gratitude to Cynthia Bourgeault, Lynn C.
Bauman, and Ward J. Bauman for their research and illumination,
I discover that there may be more to the teachings of Jesus than
I had been taught. Bourgeault says Jesus is a wisdom teacher,
teaching the perennial wisdom of the transformation of human
consciousness.[44] The *Gospel of Thomas* suggests that Jesus just may
be calling us to discover the kingdom of God within, calling us
home to our true self. A treasure indeed: Jesus, wisdom teacher,
leading us to the possibility and process of self-awakening to the
divine within.

Studying and engaging the newly-discovered Nag Hammadi
gospels, I have found that some of the teachings feel strange and
confusing, yet also raise many deep questions that intuitively feel
full of wisdom, illuminating the path of following Jesus with

heart and soul as a practice, as a way of seeing and being. Viewing the wisdom sayings from the contemplative lens of the heart brings deep, inner soul movement. For me, the *Gospel of Thomas* speaks to the contemplative Christian community—both then and now—and it is why I was drawn to use some of the *Gospel of Thomas* sayings of Jesus in the YogaMass liturgy. Interestingly, only in this post-modern time have we been given—by God's grace—Christian gospels that address a more contemplative approach and path of inner awakening to following Jesus that so many Christians are hungry for...and that so many are willing to leave their Christian faith to find.

This flight from Christianity deeply disturbs me, because my faith walk with Jesus Christ has transformed my life—he is my teacher and my path to God. I want others to know the Christ I know. It is not necessary to "leave" the Christian faith to find the way of contemplative spiritual practices that take us deep into the heart of God. The contemplative path of meditation and yoga is a direct path to God. The contemplative path is the path of Christianity that speaks most to me, a path that each may embrace. YogaMass is a very intentional offering for people to experience the depth of Christ's teachings on a personal and intimate level, and to absorb his teachings—a path that calls us to take his perspective and make it ours, completely and wholly—in our bones, our tissues, our minds, our hearts, our souls, and our spirits.

I sense a sympathetic string with the teachings of the ancient yogis. A look at the ancient teachings of yoga, the Western Canonical scriptures, and the Eastern Canon of scriptures may shine a new light on our own paths of self-discovery. Gleaning perspectives from these three sources is for me a three-legged school of inquiry that has become a profound study into the true meaning of Jesus' contemplative wisdom teachings and the realization of the kingdom of God within. What I have learned thus far is that without question, Jesus reached and embodied the highest state of consciousness as a human being. He walked the path of complete self-emptying of ego and attachments, willingly giving himself as a vessel for God's grace and love to be shared with the world, and ultimately taking a stand for love at any cost—even death.

## Discovery of the True Self

The Christian contemplative tradition emphasizes finding the True Self and releasing the False Self or the ego. Carl Jung believed that we have an ego, which represents the conscious mind comprised of thoughts, memories and emotions—of all that a person is aware of. The Ego is what helps us make sense of everything we have ever experienced, and it is what defines our identity and who we are. The ego, according to Jung, is the False Self; our True Self is not our ego. Our True Self is who we *really* are, both the known and the unknown. How we perceive ourselves is seen through the Ego, but our True Self is much more.

I find Richard Rohr's explanation of the False Self to be useful:

> Your 'false' self is how you define yourself outside of love, relationship, or divine union. After you have spent many years building this separate, egoic self, with all its labels and habits, you are very attached to it. And why wouldn't you be? It's all you know. To move beyond this privately concocted identity naturally feels like losing or dying....If you do not learn the art of dying and letting go early, you will hold onto your False Self far too long.

It was Thomas Merton, the Cistercian monk, who first suggested the use of the term *False Self.* He did this to clarify for many Christians the meaning of Jesus' central and oft-repeated teaching that we must die to ourselves, or 'lose ourselves to find ourselves.' (Mark 8:35) This quote has caused much havoc and pushback in Christian history because it sounds negative and ascetical, and it was usually interpreted as an appeal to punish the body. But its intent is personal liberation, not self-punishment.[45]

Dying to the False Self is not synonymous with dying to the body and projecting a negative image onto our bodies. The body is part of an integrated, greater whole, the Self that includes much more even than our physical body, but our psychological and emotional body as we understand in the West. And as understood in the East, the body also includes our energy bodies as well. The science of Yoga teaches us that the body is much more integrated and complex than we understand in the West. Dying to the False Self implies dying to a perspective of the body that only values its appearance and not its inherent value as an integrated part of the whole human being. For us personally and collectively, discovering, understanding, and valuing this body as a vehicle for the soul to experience God is an act of self-love.

Being human is a spiritual endeavor that includes having experiences of daily life in this body. Richard Rohr explains this well:

"We still think of ourselves as mere humans trying desperately to become "spiritual," when the Christian revelation was precisely that you are already spiritual ("in God"), and your difficult but necessary task is to learn to become human."[46]

When I am on my mat, I am completely human and spiritual, one hundred percent experiencing the Sun Salutation flow of yoga *asanas* that awakens me to remember who I am and to fully experience what I am feeling. My body, my mind, my soul, my spirit, and my breath work in tandem, reconnecting me to the experience of life in the present moment. It is in this experience that I feel fully alive, again. As Donna Fahri, yoga teacher and author, so wisely puts it, "Yoga is a technology for arriving in this present moment."[47]

## An Integral Approach with Yoga as a Spiritual Practice

The transformation of body, mind, soul, and spirit is the work of Yoga. As Christians, we would add that it is the Holy Spirit leading us in this transformation. When we sit for meditation or go to our mats for movement and breath, we inherently feel this transformation happening. We go without expectation of any specific results or breakthroughs, only with a simple awareness that we are intentionally participating in a sacred act of being still and breathing, or moving with awareness of our sacred breath.

Perhaps just as Christianity is being squeezed into changes and new emergent expressions of thought, ritual and belief, postmodern perspectives are similarly influencing the philosophical thought of the yogic system. We only need look at the varied expressions and flavors of yoga postures and practices being taught in the West to see the expansion of the flourishing emergence.

Over the millennia, philosophers of yoga have expanded and refined the philosophy and practice. Bede Griffiths, a British-born Benedictine monk and priest of the 20th century, and also a yogi, compliments the contributions of Sri Aurobindo of Calcutta in developing an integral yoga in his lifetime (1872-1950) that values life, matter, history and personality with a wonderful synthesis based on the Vedanta (a school of Indian philosophy):

In Aurobindo, the values of being and becoming, of spirit and matter, of the One and the many, of the eternal and the temporal, of the universal and the individual, of the personal God and the absolute Godhead, are integrated in a vision of the whole....

In Christian yoga [as Sri Aurobindo referred to the practice of yoga for Christians] the body and soul are to be transfigured by the divine life and to participate in the divine consciousness. There is a descent of the Spirit into matter and a corresponding ascent, by which matter is transformed by the indwelling power of the Spirit and the body is transfigured.... There must be a movement of ascent to pure consciousness, a detachment from all the moods of nature, a realization of the Self in its eternal Ground beyond space and time. But then there must also be a movement of decent, by which Spirit enters into the depths of matter and raises it to a new mode of existence, in which it becomes the medium of a spiritual consciousness.

For a Christian, this has already taken place in the resurrection of Christ.... This is the cosmic drama, this transformation of nature, of matter and the body, so as to become the outward form of the divine Spirit, the body of the Lord. And this transformation is taking place in our own bodies.[48]

The possibility of God's Spirit within our own bodies is real for Griffiths. Yogis know the soul is within our body in this life, longing to touch the divine. What if the church could teach about this personal transformation of the indwelling Spirit of God that is grounded in our bodies? What if the church could help everyone discover this truth for him or herself? How might we embrace the teachings of Christ differently to experience the ascent of pure consciousness personally and collectively? Communities of faith can engage these teachings to raise the community to a higher level of self-realization of God's presence among them and within them as we do at Grace Episcopal Church Houston. I experience deep joy when members in the community begin to explore and discern the truth of their own being, feeling safe and loved. Each of us is invited and then called to discover this life-giving transformation for spiritual awakening.

## The Path Through the Church

Jesus said, "Ask and you shall receive, seek and you shall find." In our post, post-modern age we are asking, and we are discovering, the truths of our own existence. We are discovering how imperfectly perfect we are, human and yet made of the same Spirit of God. Those who describe themselves as "spiritual but not religious" are changing the landscape of spiritual community. From 2007 to 2014, according to Pew Research Center, the Religious "nones"—those who describe themselves as atheists or agnostics and those who say they have no particular religion—grew from 16% of Americans to roughly 23% of the US adult population.[49] Of the "nones" surveyed in 2014, 40% said they feel a deep sense of spiritual peace and well-being at least weekly.[50]

Spirituality and community service are no longer dependent on a village church, temple, or synagogue as they once were. Non-profit organizations provide many ways to serve those in need. Virtual communities gather on the Internet for spiritual teachings, spiritual direction, yoga instruction, and so much more. Our global communication network has opened communication across religions and given people new language, new concepts, new ways of viewing a global community and global consciousness. It seems to me that transformation of the human race into a community of greater spiritual consciousness is happening before our very eyes, along with an equally powerful force to keep consciousness from rising (hatred, prejudice, bullying, violence, war, and mass weapons of destruction, to name a few). The role of the church must be—and is needed now more than ever—to raise the consciousness of the Christian community, to bring Christ Consciousness and the love that flows from it into the realm of possibility and practice.

The church exists as a community that seeks to reconcile all people back to God and into unity with each other in Christ. As the community of followers of Jesus, we meet together to share in his divine life. Early Christian communities called the movement of following him "the Way." The church often emphasizes *believing in* Jesus over teaching the practice of the *Way* of Jesus. For many, the belief system doesn't connect with the experience of God. My experiences in talking with the "spiritual but not religious" is that they want to experience and to "live" their spirituality, to discover divine presence for themselves, and to see it in all of creation, across religions and cultures, across the animal kingdom, and in Mother Earth who needs our help. Bede Griffiths encourages us to see that this divine life is "present everywhere and in everything, in every religion and in every human heart."[51]

The church, now more than ever, can offer Christians the opportunity to awaken to the experience of the kingdom within. The church, as difficult as it may be for some, is also being called into a new relationship with people and truths of other faith traditions. Beyond the process of dialogue for greater understanding of each other's viewpoints and beliefs, the church may soon discover that faithful people of all religions are seeking this same divine life, walking the path of divine realization, desiring to embrace each other as brothers and sisters on this planet. Just as human beings are evolving gradually over time, and adapting quickly (and necessarily!) to the societal and technological changes, so too must the church evolve over time, and adapt to modern-day changes pressing upon us all. It is the message and not the messenger that matters; it is the principles that are universal. That is not to say that devotion to the teacher who brings us to God is not important; it certainly is and may be the spiritual work of a lifetime. But ultimately the messenger brings us to a realization or truth that we ourselves must learn on our soul journey.

The gift the church can give to the world is to offer an experience of the path to discovering the kingdom of God within, holding up Jesus Christ as a mirror and a guide. This path of Jesus has always been here, but the treasure has been hidden in buried scrolls. Having now been unearthed after nearly 2,000 years, it is imperative that we bring this path of inner awakening into the light for all to discover. Just as when the sun shines at noon overhead, and there are no longer shadows, we must do our shadow work and bring the full teachings of Jesus into the light and into the world. It is our role, as followers of Jesus who loved his friends to the end, to live into the eternal Truth of Christ and to shine His light for others to not only see, but as the late Unity movement theologian Eric Butterworth said, "to see from within that light." To see from within the light, we must *become* that light ourselves.

# 5

## Wholeness and Union –
## Goals of the Spiritual Life

Mary arose, then, embracing them all and began to address
them as her brothers and sisters saying: "Do not weep
and grieve nor let your hearts remain in doubt, for his
grace will be with all of you, sustaining and protecting
you. Rather, let us give praise to his greatness which has
prepared us so that we might become true human beings.
                          –*The Gospel of Mary, Dialogue Two*[52]

### Union with God

The path to a life in God is both an outward and an inward
journey. Outwardly, we find God in our midst—in the church,
among the people, in nature, and everywhere. We find God in
the most unlikely of places: in the hearts and bodies of the sick
and the hungry, the helpless and the poor. That's why we discover
along the way that we need to serve in some way those whom
God places on our path. The outward journey takes us to the
church, to hospitals, to soup kitchens, to community gardens,
and to visit the homebound. The inward journey takes us into
our own bodies and our hearts, to find God speaking to us in our
innermost depths. The outward journey we walk with others; the
inward journey is ours alone to walk with God.

Both are paths to the kingdom of God, the vision of God
that Jesus worked for and wished to lead us to experience. He

taught us to pray, "Thy kingdom come." The kingdom of God is a vision at first we almost cannot imagine: it is utopia, it is the Garden of Eden before the fall, and it is heaven on earth. We imagine re-entry into the Garden as the experience of walking back into the kingdom of God, and it feels so unattainable. As our spiritual journey progresses, we eventually come to know that the kingdom of God is union with God in our innermost beings.

Union with God comes from knowing our True Self and returning to the presence of God. The purpose of religion is to provide a vehicle, a set of tools, values, and beliefs that help people move toward God on the path to union with God. As a priest, I am called to lead people in the process of transformation, in the experience of healing, forgiveness, and integrating mind, body, soul, and spirit so that the discovery of being in union with God in our innermost being becomes a real possibility.

Initially as I develop relationships with people, my hope is to first help them believe that they are loved and worthy to be loved. This is often a lifetime's work. Only when a person believes he or she is worthy to be loved can God's love fully permeate their entire being. The heart and mind have to be open and ready to receive this truth. If every girl and boy, and adult, who is searching for something or someone to fill the longing in their hearts could know deep within that they are worthy of love, of God's love, simply because they exist, with no strings attached, I believe there would be much less suffering. So much time would not be wasted searching for the love that has been—and is—there all along. We could then begin the process of transformation for a life filled with receiving and giving love, discovering that God is present in and among all people, and to serving others, simply for the sake of love.

Many Christians focus on heaven as a place where we go after death. But heaven doesn't have to be simply about what happens to us after we die. It is when we become completely integrated, completely whole, that we discover heaven on earth. This is the true meaning of salvation: wholeness and integration. We pray in the words of Jesus, "Thy kingdom come, thy will be done, on earth as in heaven." Do we really understand the present moment inherent in that prayer? It is not a prayer about the future, it is a prayer for now, for the present moment, for the time we are living: for this day, this hour, this moment, this breath. My daily prayer: Holy God, your kingdom come, now, live around me and in me...in the space, in the experience, and beyond this experience, simply in the faces of everyone I meet and in the silence within the cave of my heart.

The evolution of spirituality must be that spirituality becomes a conscious vehicle for personal transformation and awakening into the presence of the divine. In my own journey, I have delightedly found deep congruence in the Eastern gospels of transformation and their resonance with the science of yogic practices as sympathetic strings.

Paramahansa Yogananda, yoga master and spiritual teacher of the early twentieth century in the United States, describes the parallel of this teaching of personal transformation with yoga, since the word "yoke" in the original Greek and the word "yoga" both derive from the Sanskrit root *yuj*, signifying "union." Jesus said, "Take my yoke upon you, and learn from me, for I am gentle and lowly in heart, and you will find rest for your souls" (Matthew 11:29). Yogananda describes the meaning of this teaching of Jesus:

> "In oneness with the infinite Christ intelligence, Jesus lovingly urged all spiritual aspirants to 'Come unto me' (the Christ Consciousness) and 'Take my yoke upon you'—follow the step-by-step methods of self-discipline that lead to Christ Consciousness and that assure ultimate liberation in God's kingdom."[53]

The *Gospel of Thomas* also points us to move into a state of wholeness from every layer of our being. I use this saying of Yeshua from the *Gospel of Thomas*, Logion 70, in the YogaMass liturgy:

> "When you give birth to that which is within yourself; what you bring forth will save you. If you possess nothing within, that absence will destroy you."

## The Wisdom Teaching of the *Gospel of Thomas* Logion 70: The Divine Within

Self-discovery, birth, creativity, and healing: this is a path of integration and wholeness. I am intrigued by this saying—its femininity, its invitation, its challenge. This wisdom teaching of Logion 70 resonates with me on five unique levels.

First, it speaks to the divine within and the inherent goodness within us that God wants us to bring forth in our full capacity of being human. For that which is within you is sufficient to save you. What is within that has that much value? What absence can have so much power that it will destroy you? The contemplative spiritual path is the discovery of that which is within you, the very presence of God, the divine spark—and that discovery is life changing and transformative. Can you remember a time when you just felt right with the world, and everything was exactly as it should be? When your life seemed to be flowing just as naturally as nature flows?

Second, it speaks to creativity desiring to be born and fully expressed. Bringing forth what your heart wants to say is one of the greatest gifts we can give ourselves. Expressing your inner light and voice is an act of self-compassion. And God just may be calling your voice (expressed in art, poetry, music, literature, or any creative outlet, which can even be your life's work) to come out and into the world, for the greater good. Or could it be that God is calling forth your voice and your creation for your own healing? No matter the level of good that it creates, your expression is healing, and bringing it forth is an act of creating wholeness.

Third, in Jungian terms, this Logion 70 wisdom teaching speaks to the unconscious, what Carl Jung calls the shadow. The shadow represents instinctual energies that are repressed and reside in the unconscious. These energies are not part of conscious awareness, and bringing them into consciousness is the work of integrating parts of our personality into wholeness, bringing them into the light. In spiritual direction work, I help people discover their rejected self, the self that has become hidden in the darkness, and bring their repressed energies forward to be expressed. Hidden or repressed energies will eventually come out through their own volition anyway, and usually not in healthy ways. Giving birth to the shadow, acknowledging and expressing it, releases its hold on us and creates greater inner balance. Thus, by doing shadow work we are liberated and set free.

This Wisdom teaching speaks to the necessity of doing this work of healing repressed emotions and memories. We do this in the Western world through various healing modalities, including psychotherapy, spiritual direction, and dream work, to name a few. In Eastern philosophy, yoga is one way to address the repressed and stored emotions and memories in the body, and yoga assists in releasing blockages on many levels, in the physical, emotional, and subtle bodies.

Fourth, this Wisdom teaching speaks to the process of attaining self-knowledge and the processes of individuation or autonomy and integration to become whole. For Jung, developing a balance of the archetypal energies of the inner female and male of our psyches, as Jung defines them (the *anima* and the *animus*), is the path to integration and wholeness. In spiritual direction, I help my directees to understand the stereotypes they are embracing in their lives, to recognize the archetypes that impact the way they view themselves and others, to reflect on how they are embracing or resisting spiritual energies in their lives, and to balance the masculine and feminine attitudes, perspectives, and behaviors within themselves. (I'll be addressing the *anima* and the *animus* more, later in this chapter.)

Finally, Logion 70 also speaks to the process of discovery of the human soul in our deepest, truest, divine nature. It calls us to not be led by the ego, or the False Self, and to bring forth the True Self, the infinite Christ Consciousness that was incarnate in Jesus. Mary Magdalene expressed this goal so clearly as a teaching Jesus gave to her: to become "a true human being." "Giving birth to that which is within yourself" speaks to self-affirmation, creativity, expression, self-discovery, inner healing, individuation, integration, and awareness of God within. It also resonates with the yogic *chakra* system (which I will describe in more detail later in Chapter 7). To attain self-knowledge and discover our True Self is the path to salvation, and the Christian path according to Mary Magdalene in the *Gospel of Mary* is to become a true human. This infers that there is much more to living in a sacred way than we have been taught to believe is possible.

## The Meaning of Salvation is Wholeness

Salvation is a Christian doctrine that focuses on ethics or right behavior, and the insistence on right belief. We usually think of salvation as being made right with God, as being "saved by grace" as St. Paul described in his letter to the community in Ephesus: "For by grace you have been saved through faith, and this is not your own doing; it is the gift of God" (Ephesians 2:8). Grace is freely given through God's amazing love, and the gift is that we don't have to earn grace. You may have experienced grace when an unsuspecting person says to you exactly what you needed to hear at that moment of confusion, isolation, or desperation. God's amazing grace may come to you through a mystical experience of God, or simply through another human being's act of love. It's all grace. I have come to know that even—and especially—*breath* is grace.

For many, salvation is about what happens to us after we die. If we are "saved," we will go to heaven; if not, we're in trouble. But this narrow interpretation lacks the beauty of the present moment, of how we are living life right now. To discover the true meaning of salvation, we look to the Bible for instruction. Salvation is deliverance, redemption, being rescued, being set free. In the life of the Hebrew people, God is the one who delivers both the community and the individual. The personal experience of salvation is expressed in the Psalter and in the New Testament:

> "Make me to know your ways, O Lord; teach me your paths.
>
> Lead me in your truth, and teach me, for you are the God of my salvation; for you I wait all day long." (Psalm 25:4-5)
>
> "And Mary said, "My soul magnifies the Lord, and my spirit rejoices in God my Savior, for he has looked with favor on the lowliness of his servant. Surely, from now on all generations will call me blessed; for the Mighty One has done great things for me, and holy is his name." (Luke 1:46-49, excerpt of Mary's *Magnificat*)

In looking to the original Greek in the New Testament for guidance, we find that the salvation is "wholeness," coming from the Greek word *soteria* (meaning salvation, wholeness) and the

Greek word *soter* (meaning savior, one who makes whole). If salvation is wholeness, it benefits us to consider a holistic approach to our entire self: the body, the rational mind, the emotions, the psyche, and the spiritual health of the soul and spirit. Well-being is essential to obtaining wholeness. Relationships between each of these components drive the overall health and well-being of an individual, and for that matter, a collective group of people as well. Wholeness is multi-dimensional.

When physical well-being is sought, it is critical to hear what Dr. Candace Pert, neuroscientist and pharmacologist, famously stated about the relationship between the body and the mind: "Your body is your subconscious mind. Our physical body can be changed by the emotions we experience."[54] We store all of our memories and our emotions in our bodies, and physical well-being requires that we address our psychological state and emotions, that we work through them, that we heal them, so that they are no longer held in our bodies in harmful ways. Healing and wholeness occur when balance is attained. Dr. Pert explains the physiology of this:

> A feeling sparked in our mind—or body—will translate as a peptide being released somewhere. [Organs, tissues, skin, muscle and endocrine glands], they all have peptide receptors on them and can access and store emotional information. This means the emotional memory is stored in many places in the body, not just or even primarily, in the brain. You can access emotional memory anywhere in the peptide/receptor network, in any number of ways. I think unexpressed emotions are literally lodged in the body. The real true emotions that need to be expressed are in the body, trying to move up and be expressed and thereby integrated, made whole, and healed.[55]

The state of wholeness is in part a function of expression of emotion, healing, and transformation of consciousness. Dr. Pert's work on Mind-Body medicine affirms the linkage between our conscious and subconscious mind and their effect on the body. Memories of wounding and hurts, sorrows and disappointments, can linger for a lifetime, keeping one stuck and unable to move beyond the past. The inability to forgive and release painful memories keeps one from fully engaging in the new life that Jesus promises: "I came that they may have life, and have it abundantly" (John 10:10b). Attention to the body through the practice of yoga helps to release stuck emotions and stagnant energy in the body in a gradual process of the healing of these painful memories. Yoga postures do more than stretch us and keep us flexible; they also offer physical and emotional healing in deeper ways than we can imagine. As memories stored deep in our bodies are released, we can finally let go of the emotional hold they have on us. We are finally set free from the patterns associated with these memories, and we are able to move on in a more healthy and holistic approach to life.

## Wholeness in the Human Being

A holistic approach to healing also includes the psychological integration of Carl Jung's masculine and feminine archetypal energies of the psyche, known as *anima* and *animus*. These archetypal energies are universal, repeating patterns of thought and action that appear in people in every continent, country, ethnicity, and gender. Both masculine and feminine energies are present within each of us, although as archetypal energies they are not gender specific. Each influences our personalities and behaviors in both positive and negative ways if they are under- or overdeveloped. The goal of psychological wholeness is to cultivate a balance of *anima* and *animus*.

In general, men have an underdeveloped relationship with their *anima* (feminine energy), and women have an underdeveloped relationship with their *animus* (masculine energy). Consequently, psychological wholeness requires women to befriend their *animus* (masculine energy) and men to befriend their *anima* (feminine energy.) As both men and women develop psychological and spiritual maturity, they achieve a greater balance and integration of these masculine and feminine energies. Salvation, in Christian terms, incorporates the process of integrating the *anima* and the *animus* for psychological development, balance and wholeness, which also leads to higher spiritual maturity. As Yeshua taught in the *Gospel of Thomas* to those desiring to be on their way into the kingdom:

> "When you are able to make two become one, the inside like the outside, and the outside like the inside, the higher like the lower, so that a man is no longer male, and a woman, female, but male and female become a single whole. When you are able to fashion an eye to replace an eye, and form a hand in place of a hand, or a foot for a foot, making one image supersede another—then you will enter in" (Logion 22).

The masculine archetypal energy of the *animus* is symbolized by potency, power, focus, discernment, differentiation, and penetration—all masculine attributes in his phallus quality. These energies are further reflected by the ability to articulate and express ideas and thoughts using words, language, and logic, based on the Greek word Logos, λόγος, which means word, reason, and logic in its original meaning. When a man develops the unconscious feminine energies, the *anima*, within himself, he achieves wholeness, balance, and health of the psyche. A healthy *anima* in a man reveals qualities of sensitivity, tenderness, vulnerability, openness, nurturing, creativity, emotional expression, and collaboration. Sadly, the archetypal feminine qualities in a man are not traditionally valued by Western society, even though development of these qualities is necessary for spiritual and psychological wholeness. Tragically, in the West, a general proclivity toward the dark side of the masculine energies of the *animus*—survival, exclusivity, possessiveness, jealousy, and punitive actions—not only exists, but is culturally desired and required, perpetuated by societal fear-based messages, often preventing men from exploring and embracing the feminine archetypal qualities within themselves.

The feminine archetypal energy of the *anima* is symbolized by openness, receptivity, adaptability, inclusivity, multi-tasking, and retention—all attributes of the feminine in her womb-like quality. These energies are further reflected by the non-rational desire to connect, relate or create, based on the Greek word Eros. Eros is not really about eroticism as culture teaches us; Eros is about experience and sensuality. When a woman develops her unconscious masculine energies, the *animus* within herself, she achieves psychological and spiritual wholeness, balance, and health. A healthy *animus* in a woman reveals three primary qualities: focus, discernment, and differentiation. These qualities are essential to bringing balance and wholeness in a woman. They can also be described in terms of qualities of strength, fortitude, autonomy, independence, assertiveness, competitiveness, freedom of expression, and teamwork.

Women have assumed more roles in the working world over the last 70 years, increasing their personal independence and autonomy; these qualities are being developed and exercised by women in many varied ways. However, if a woman overdevelops her masculine energies to survive in a "man's world," she may unknowingly bring about the dark side of the masculine energy, which only further perpetuates the global dilemma of an exclusive mindset and mechanisms that support an overly competitive, fearful, and survival mode mentality.

The wholeness the spiritual life seeks is to bring a woman's and a man's feminine and masculine qualities into balance. For Jung, growth towards wholeness ("individuation") implies an acceptance and integration of the *animus* and *anima* archetypes. In psychological terms, the *animus*, or masculine energy, is solar, and the *anima*, or feminine energy, is lunar. There is a correlation of these energies in yogic practices: the channel systems or Sanskrit *nadis*.

Dr. David Frawley, Western-born teacher and author on the Vedic tradition, describes these channels in terms of nature: "Just as there are channels in the body, so external nature is filled with various channels—from rivers and streams to currents of energy in intergalactic space."[56] According to the science of yoga, each person has a lunar, feminine and cooling energy, and a solar, masculine and heating energy. Yogic practices seek to balance these energies in the physical body and what yoga calls the subtle body (mind-*prana* field) for wholeness and spiritual development, as David Frawley describes:

> "Once the flow becomes completely liberated, it merges us back into the ocean of consciousness that dwells within the heart; the free flow becomes one with silence and stillness."[57]

This balance, integration, and wholeness are what both yogic and psychological-spiritual practices seek to create. Jesus in the Eastern *Gospel of Philip* seems to suggest this very integration as a goal of the spiritual life (Analogue 41):

> There are both male and female spirits, which at heart are unclean and impure. Male spirits seek to mate with souls that inhabit a female form,

and female spirits seek an unequal relationship with a male form. So no one, then, is able to escape being seized by their compulsions if they have not received both the power of the male and the female in equal balance. It is in the iconic Bridal Chamber, where the bride is united with the bridegroom that this balance is attained.[58]

In Jungian terms, men and women seeking to develop the unconscious part of their psychology undergo "shadow" work to become more personally healed, whole and fulfilled. Being whole means we actually don't need another person to complete us: we can become whole within ourselves, with God's help. We become fully capable of being in a healthy, mutually-supportive relationship when we are psychologically whole. I remember the movie where Tom Cruise tells the woman he loves in that famous kitchen scene, "You complete me," and women all over the world watching this movie *melted* hearing those words—because we all want to feel that kind of love and connection and sense of being needed. But the truth is we don't really need another human being to "complete" us. The truth is, no one else *can* complete us: wholeness is inner work. Another human being whom we love dearly may complement us and help us to completely live into our humanity and spirituality, and this is the nature of human relationships at their best. This is friendship, partnership, and the theological basis for marriage as a sacrament. Another human being—a partner, a spouse, a soul mate—can help us become whole "within" by helping us heal, by being a mirror for us to see ourselves as others see us, and by journeying with us to become whole. All of this is possible only by love, by being both the lover and the beloved.

The spiritual life is the journey to becoming whole and integrated. For Christians, we are sealed by the power of God's Holy Spirit in Baptism and invited to live into that reality of

Spirit connection throughout our lives. We arrive at a point in life where we want to become fully engaged in life and in our "human being-ness," as spiritual beings. At this point, salvation becomes real, and it isn't simply a term that refers to whether or not we have done enough right things to be able to go to a designated place when we die, like "heaven." Salvation is really about wholeness, and we can obtain this state of being any time, for today and for eternity. The truth is, our souls are never apart from God, except at the hand of our own free will when we do things that lead us away from the heart of God.

Ram Dass coined the phrase "Be here now" in his classic book by the same title, as a reminder to find that wholeness, that peace and groundedness within us. It sounds so simple, and yet so profound. To "be here now" is also available to us in terms of awareness from within the body, as I spoke of earlier. In terms of spiritual experience, when all is right with our soul, when our soul is aligned with God, we can be in the present moment, living fully right now, in God's presence. Eternity will come, all in God's time. It is only in the present moment, in these bodies, that we can take action and live wholly and complete, aligned with God and with our own hearts. That is how I choose to live, all the time.

## The Science of Human Experience and Realization of the Divine

I'm probably like many people that have misunderstandings about yoga. Like many others, I originally thought yoga was a religion, or that it was based in the beliefs of Hinduism and Buddhism. I believed that yoga was a religion of foreign gods, and therefore off-limits for me, a Christian. God spoke to Moses on Mt. Sinai, saying explicitly, "Thou shalt have no other gods before me" (Exodus 20:3). However, after affirming how good

I felt when moving through the yoga postures as exercise, I did my research and learned that in actuality, yoga is a *science*. Yoga is the science of the human experience. It addresses all aspects of a person: the physical, vital, mental, emotional, psychic, and spiritual. Yoga is the science of "right living," and intended to be incorporated into daily life as a practice, a way of "being," so that one can ultimately realize union with the divine. Thus, yoga is not a religion, but it can be a spiritual path.

Yoga is a "science" because from its inception, the earliest yogis were methodically "experimenting" with the practices and techniques that helped one gain intuitive knowledge about union with the divine. Yoga as a science is also a spiritual experience, because our spiritual life cannot be separated from our minds and our bodies. The late Swami Satyananda Saraswati, yoga teacher and founder of the Divine Life Society, describes the precise method of yoga as a spiritual practice: "This unity or joining is described in spiritual terms as the union of the individual consciousness with the universal consciousness."[59] Swami Satyananda adds, "On a more practical level, yoga is a means of balancing and harmonizing the body, mind, and emotions."[60] This balance that can be achieved with the practice of yoga results in a wholeness and sense of well-being that is experienced and enjoyed both on and off the mat. One of my yoga teachers describes the "union" as a marriage between body and breath. Clearly, the layers of union are multi-dimensional, just like the layered meanings of salvation as wholeness.

Historically, yoga originated before religious language, but it was religious tradition that helped give it shape and form through human methods of communication. Swami Satyananda offers an informative history of yoga that predates most known civilizations and describes how yoga arose and evolved through mythical tradition and religious language:

Yoga arose at the beginning of human civilization when humankind first realized their spiritual potential and began to evolve techniques to develop it.... It developed as part of the tantric civilization that existed in India more than ten thousand years ago. In archaeological excavations made in the Indus Valley, now in modern Pakistan, statues have been found depicting deities...performing various *asanas* and practicing meditation. These ruins were once the dwelling place of people who lived in the pre-vedic age before the Aryan civilization started to flourish in the Indus subcontinent. According to the mythical tradition, Shiva is said to be the founder of yoga...and is considered to be the symbol or embodiment of supreme consciousness. Parvati... regarded as the mother of the whole universe, represents supreme knowledge, will and action, and is responsible for all creation.[61]

While it might seem unsettling that ancient deities were depicted as performing *asanas*, this need not threaten Christian beliefs. With all intentions of respect to the religious traditions of ancient civilizations and other faith traditions today, the deities are depictions of their God (and gods and goddesses) teaching humans how to be both spiritual and human. Outside of the land and culture of the Judeo-Christian people, we might better understand (and celebrate) that for them, Shiva and Parvati are two manifestations of God. While Christians believe in one God, we also have a way of viewing God as a Triune God: God the Father, God the Son, and God the Holy Spirit.

All faith traditions and religions use their language and concepts to make sense of the experience of God. As medieval Italian philosopher and theologian Thomas Aquinas taught in his Doctrine of Analogy, we use experiential language to try to speak of the truth of God. God is ultimately beyond language, beyond any form that humans may need to find expression of the ultimate and mysterious Truth. What is intriguing and exciting to me is that the ancient expression of their gods *over 10,000 years ago* recognized yoga *asanas* and meditation as paths to the divine.

Some yogic traditions believe that yoga was a divine gift revealed to ancient sages so that humankind could have the opportunity to realize its divine nature.[62] The Vedas, for example, were written as the primary texts of Hinduism, with the oldest, the *Rig Veda*, composed about 1500 B.C., and codified about 600 B.C. The *Bhagavad Gita*, written somewhere in the 5th to 2nd century BCE, provides instruction on daily living and the spiritual path to union with God. *Bhagavad Gita* means "Song of the Spirit," the divine communion of truth-realization between man and Creator, the teachings of Spirit through the soul, that should be sung unceasingly. The Gita is set in a narrative framework of a dialogue between the guide and charioteer Lord Krishna and Arjuna (a symbol for all who would seek God) as he is on the battlefield. The timeless message of the *Bhagavad Gita* does not refer only to a historical battle, but to the cosmic and inner conflict between good and evil. It is a powerful message that helps illumine the path for the spiritual seeker, using the science of yoga as a path to union with God. The *Bhagavad Gita* is studied in yoga communities for its yogic ideals and framework for spiritual progress.

## A Greater Truth

Some may wonder why a Christian could or would study religious texts or philosophies outside of their own culture or religious tradition. In my personal experience, Christians who participate in study of interfaith texts and dialogue with other religious communities can gain rich insights that take us deeper into our own religious understanding and beliefs.

In the early stage of my priesthood journey, I studied the early church Patristic fathers' writings, I studied the saints of the church, and I studied the writings about the women in early Christianity. I was struck by the silence of the women in the narrative, and was left hungry to know more. What about the lives of Mary Magdalene, Mother Mary, Salome, and Thecla that could inform my own faith journey? I studied the non-canonical *Gospel of Mary* to hear what she had to say about Jesus. I was strongly grounded in my faith in Jesus, and yet I knew there was more to the story than what was being told. Elisabeth Schüssler Fiorenza, feminist theologian and professor, named the process of discovering the silent voices in Scripture "exegesis of the silence." This concept empowered me to continue on my journey of discovery with imagination and questions that couldn't be answered readily by the faith stories handed down through my tradition.

In my own life, I was tending to the spiritual calling of finding and speaking my voice, resulting in my heart resonating even more strongly with the millions of women whose voices had never been heard. Along the way, I began to intuit that I was resonating with the voice of the feminine aspect of God known by ancient civilizations. I became aware of these goddesses whose voices and wisdom were silenced when God became male in the evolution of the Abrahamic tradition, which is my inherited tradition. I found myself standing on the ruins of Temples of Athena and Artemis in Greece and Turkey on a pilgrimage in St. Paul's footsteps, and my heart felt a resonance, a deep gladness, and a deep longing for the divine feminine that touched me to my core in ways I could not explain or understand at the time. As the questions became more urgent in my head and my heart, practicing yoga on my mat helped me to daily settle me down into a state of "it's okay-ness."

I remain hopeful that a greater awareness of the narratives spanning all civilizations will contribute to the global rise of human consciousness, and humankind will progress biologically, psychologically, socially, culturally, and spiritually with a more balanced approach to our understanding of God and our interconnectedness. I choose to contribute to the re-emergence of the divine feminine, the feminine aspect of God, and her re-emergence within humanity, so that she continues to rise from the ashes, taking her role once again as a valued voice in creation. The silenced voices must be heard in new ways, speaking through the wisdom traditions across all religions. I trust that in time, the voice of Divine Wisdom, *Sophia*, will ring out with new understandings for the healing of our collective hearts and bodies, and the rising consciousness will become available to all, including those who follow the Way of Jesus. For without her voice, we will not individually and collectively achieve balance, harmony, and peace.

However unsettling, leaving the safe boundaries of the spiritually familiar for an even greater truth and knowledge has been the path of spiritual growth for me. The retired Episcopal Bishop in the United States, John Shelby Spong, while his views may be controversial to some, gave me a new understanding of the journey of exploration and expansion as a path to discovering a new truth beyond what one tradition teaches:

> "The evidence that God, understood theistically, is dying or is perhaps already dead is overwhelming. I [Spong] define the theistic God as a being, supernatural in power, dwelling outside this world and invading the world periodically to accomplish the divine will."[63]

Bishop Spong isn't saying that God is dead, but that the image we have placed on God may be shifting. It doesn't seem such a surprise that he makes the conclusion that Christianity, as we know it, must change or die. Christ Consciousness as a possibility for all creation is moving across the waters at an unsurpassed rate. The supernatural God who dwells outside of our world and reappears only at certain times is a transcendent God that I was taught as a young child to fear (the fatherly God who watches and judges me). That fear was real for me, as for many, until I became consciously aware that God is both transcendent all the time *and* immanent all the time, both outside and within me, leading me to all truths and loving me as I grow and evolve. My God even forgives me when I miss the mark (the true definition of sin!) and come home to God and my True Self, grounded in love.

When expressing my fears of individuation into my own truth to Pittman McGehee, I was grateful for his guidance and encouragement. He validated my ever-expanding view, teaching me that my journey is precisely the path of ongoing conversion, which is one of the vows I made as a Benedictine Oblate: to continue an ongoing conversion *into the heart of God.* Instead of condemning me or questioning my faith, he reframed it for me. Rather than being unfaithful, I am being more faithful, growing into a deeper sense of the collective belonging of all and the divine within all of God's creation.

The integration of the body into worship and the creation of YogaMass are how I have dealt with my instinct of a deeper truth, and how I hope to bring others to know God as I know God. Bishop Spong goes on to say:

> The old myth of theism has lost its power and its appeal. A new myth to which we can once again be committed is not yet in place. Before the new myth can be developed, we need to understand how the old one was born, how its power was kept intact for so long, and how it has died. Perhaps then we will have a clue where to

begin our struggle to kindle once more a faith, a way of life, even a God who is not subject to the death of theism. At least that is our next step.[64]

So where now will we find our God?

## Making Room for the (Ancient) New

These are exciting times in the evolution of humanity: the interest and exploration of meditation, yoga *asanas*, and other yogic aspects are bringing us toward greater self-knowledge and experiences of mystical revelation. Historically, during periods in which reported mystical experiences were prevalent, the times devolved into "dark" periods of humanity's progress. For example, in the 15th century and into the Puritan era of the West, over nine million women and some men were burned at the stake, labeled as "witches" because of their interest in healing, herbs, creativity, and intuition. This was indeed a dark time, when the collective unconscious could not allow the creative, feminine aspect to have its rightful place in society.

By contrast, now is a time (at least in the West) when women can speak our hearts and our truth without fear of abusive retribution. Healing touch, acupressure, acupuncture, meditation, yoga, homeopathic practices, nutrition, herbal remedies, aromatherapy, and Eastern practices are becoming more and more widely accepted as alternatives and supplemental approaches to western medicine, and are practiced by men and women alike. Interestingly, as the church struggles with the rise of spiritual awareness in the West of broader perspectives of truths available to the collective, we also must admit that the healing modalities and their impact are not necessarily religious in nature; instead, they recognize and value different perspectives of the body's energy system, breath, and the connectivity of body, mind, soul, and spirit—all interrelated and inseparable.

And yet, the healing modalities are indeed *spiritual* in nature. How interesting it is that spiritual seekers are finding ways to do their soul and spirit work in ways that are not necessarily accompanied by the church or its priest. I have more to say about the personal spiritual life in relation to the need for community in Chapter 10, and thus the need for a spiritual community such as the church for awakening into and living within a higher spiritual consciousness.

Younger generations are exploring spirituality through the Internet, blogs, and social media. Communication channels that not only bring the world to our fingertips, but also spiritual teachings from the many world religions and traditions have expanded exponentially. Young people are exploring spirituality and they are often spiritual activists, embodying their spirituality in diverse ways such as helping on a mission project, a food pantry, or a community garden—or simply finding God within on their yoga mats. The church, as a physical entity, must take note—if the church is to restore its relevancy—of how spiritual seeking is changing, how these avenues of seeking are not centered in one place or house of worship, but in many places, both virtually *and* locally embodied.

Still, the church has an important purpose. Seeking a spiritual life benefits greatly from community, and church is one way to experience community and to learn and grow spiritually with others. Perhaps the hardest part about being in community is learning to love—universally and unconditionally—in spite of all the challenges inherent in any community or family system, and not giving up when something is not to your liking (notwithstanding abusive or dangerous relationships). God doesn't give up on us, and God is our guide on how to be in relationship with God and all of creation, especially each other! It's all about learning to love with a higher consciousness, also known as *agape* love.

The spiritual path often begins as a personal path for many: exploring various ways to find God, becoming aware of God's presence among and within, and opening to serve fellow human beings and the planet. Young people ask me questions in their search, and they ask me not to tell them *what* to believe but to let them discover their path for themselves. As a priest, I take the role not of an expert but rather as a spiritual guide. They take responsibility for their spiritual journey, and they know innately that *how* they live their lives matters. Young people inherently know that what happens to one affects all of us. What happens to the planet affects all of us. Many are finding truths that speak to them beyond the tradition they were born into. This is the reality of our time. Some people within organized religion are afraid of this expansive view of interconnectivity and networked approach to spirituality, and others, like me, are set free. I do not always have to be right, and opening my heart to learn wisdom from other traditions feels free and liberating.

## Fear of the Unknown

While human beings enjoy some spontaneity and uncertainty, humans in general need certainty. Our life is spent learning about how the world works and making sense of it so that it is manageable for us personally. Where there is too much unknown, there is fear. Sadly, and like many people growing up in the Christian faith, I was acculturated with a real fear of exploring (and even encountering) other faith traditions, because we were taught—and believe—Holy Scripture to be the authoritative word of God. There is an inherent certainty in this. As acceptance of people in other faith traditions grows, the saying of Jesus, "I am the way, and the truth, and the life. No one comes to the Father except through me" (John 14:6) is an especially challenging one.

Many Christians feel there is spiritual danger in encountering other traditions, even the actual people in those traditions, because they take this passage literally: it sounds as though Jesus is clearly stating that Jesus, *as the Son of God,* is the *only* way, the *only* truth and the *only* life. Many Christians fear people practicing yoga because it introduces another religion, other "gods," into one's belief system and consciousness. The late theologian and author Marcus J. Borg shed light on this fear for me in light of John 14:6:

> Is it really possible that nobody other than Christians can be saved? That the God of the universe has chosen to be known in only this one way? But within John's incarnational theology, the verse need not mean this. Incarnation means embodiment, becoming flesh. For John, just as Jesus is the Word of God become flesh and the wisdom of God become flesh, so he is 'the way' become flesh. For John, what we see in Jesus is the way—the incarnation, the embodiment, of a life radically centered in God. *This*—the *way* [emphasis added] we see in Jesus—is *the way*— [emphasis added].[65]

To remove the overlay of Jesus the man being the only Son of God—the gatekeeper to the word of God—and replace it with a deeper understanding that it is "the way" of Jesus—the embodiment of a life wholly and radically centered in God—that is the word of God, is liberating and life-giving. Personally, I try to follow Jesus every day of my life. To know that his way is my way gives my life meaning. He is my teacher and shows me the way to fully live in God's grace and flow. And yet, this is the struggle that I have, and many Christians have, that I have accepted is my path of ongoing conversion: I know that when I am on my yoga mat, I experience the divine around me and especially within me.

I get in touch with a part of me that has been deeply buried and is sweet and sacred. And how unsettling it once was, and truthfully still is at times, to feel I was betraying the belief system that I had been taught was the *only* right way. My foundation was shaking ever so gently, leaving me both unsure and yet very sure that there was a truth in this path that I must find.

This is why I remained silent about my unfolding spiritual journey for so long. As a priest, I have committed my life to bringing others to the knowledge and love of God. This commitment remains steadfast; what has been changing for me is my awareness of the expansiveness of God. As I was taught in seminary, there really are no complete words to describe God using human language. Our religious traditions give us a construct, a framework, using language to describe and worship God in God's fullness. Encountering the science of yoga and the tenets of other faith traditions in my ecumenical and interfaith relationships in ministry has expanded my view of God, of how God works in and through us—including people of different faith traditions—to bring us closer in relationship with God and each other. I sense a greater awareness of God's presence and God's movement in my life and in the lives of those around me, not trying to control outcomes but to allow God's movement to unfold among us and through us. This awareness of a more expansive, inclusive God has also made it challenging for me to stay within the language and ritual of one tradition as my heart hungers for wisdom.

In my silent struggle, I began to feel uncomfortable with some aspects of my belief system. My discomfort arose initially as my interfaith relationships expanded, and I began to see the compassionate and humble qualities of Jesus evident in people of other faith traditions (Muslims, Hindus, Sufis, Buddhists, to name a few). I'll always remember my first encounter ever with a Muslim man on the campus of The University of Texas Medical Branch at Galveston. This man, an Egyptian, Dr. Ahmed

Ahmed, was kind, a gentle spirit full of compassion, and I felt as if I was in the presence of Jesus himself. I have rarely in my life encountered that essence, his soul completely devoted to God. My struggle became more pronounced when I began exploring the transformation happening within me as a result of meditation and yoga practices. I became aware of a rising discomfort within when I offered some of the words of the Eucharistic prayer—particularly the words that involve Jesus as the "only" Son of God, making a sacrifice for me, and mankind, once and for all. In my priestly responsibilities, I say these words over the elements of bread and wine when celebrating the Eucharist. How difficult and challenging those words became for me as I struggled with the truth I was awakening to of the divine within each of us. (Stay tuned, as I have reconciled this, which I'll explain in Chapter 10 when I describe the sacred ritual, The Eucharist.) I went into deep prayer and discernment for quite a few months, and finally I reached my wit's end and knew I had to turn it over to God (which is always the answer, and I always wonder why it took me so long to get there, again). It was then that God spoke to me; another "soul movement" experience.

# ～6～

# Making the Ancient New (Again) – *Returning to Soul*

It is only at your source that you will find your destiny. Blessed are those who come to stand in their place of origination, for it is there that they will know their end—never tasting death.
—*The Gospel of Thomas, Logion 18*
(*The Luminous Gospels*, Bauman, Bauman, and Bourgeault)

In the darkness of a cold night, while my husband Gary and I were in Boulder, Colorado in the mountains with friends, I awoke in the early hours of the morning, when the earth and all of creation are still and quiet, and the energy of God's universe is powerfully pulsing. My heart was restless, and I spoke to God in prayer saying, "I really need your help. I don't know if I can do this. I don't know if I believe these words are true. Help me God." In that very moment, very clearly and succinctly, I heard these words in my heart: "Go back to the beginning." I felt as if the heavens opened up and gave me a direction, a place to explore, a sense of hope that I wasn't lost and had not fallen completely off the path. Another soul movement had just occurred within me. And it was a movement toward wholeness and union with Christ toward the way that he saw everything.

## Going Back to Walk with Jesus

So what exactly does "Go back to the beginning" mean? I see now that my inner voice was guiding me toward the right spiritual path for me at that time, and surprisingly, the divine feminine was taking her place, equally, within that path. In my initial interpretation, I clearly knew that I was to go back to the beginning and walk with Jesus as he walked on earth, in the land of Palestine and Israel, in the boat on the Sea of Galilee, on the stone streets and hills of Jerusalem. I was to be there with him where he healed people, as he felt them touch the cloak of his garment and he felt the energy leaving his body, as he ate with his friends, teaching them and laughing and enjoying their company. I felt I was to go back to the beginning, to the reality of his relationships with all the people, not just the twelve disciples but also the women who were there with him, supporting his ministry and who funded his ministry. To be clear, the women *were* there with him:

> "Soon afterwards he went on through cities and villages, proclaiming and bringing the good news of the kingdom of God. The twelve were with him, as well as some women who had been cured of evil spirits and infirmities: Mary, called Magdalene, from whom seven demons had gone out, and Joanna, the wife of Herod's steward Chuza, and Susanna, and many others, who provided for them out of their resources" (Luke 8:1-3).

The women encouraged him, provided for him, and loved him. They were no doubt healed by him, but also transformed by him. If any of you have experienced, like me, deep healing and emotional freedom in Jesus, you know the feeling: there is no going back.

Mary Magdalene was with Jesus wholeheartedly. Jesus healed her, and she stayed with him out of gratitude, out of love. She stayed with him, she supported him, and we know that because she was there with him all the way to the cross and to the tomb to anoint his body, as was the Jewish burial custom. She wouldn't have been at the cross if she didn't love him so fully and so completely. She wouldn't have come to the tomb alone as the Gospel writer John tells the story, in the early morning hours, if she didn't love him with her whole heart. I became very encouraged; going back to the beginning meant going back to understanding the life of Mary Magdalene and her spirituality and what it meant to be all in and to give her entire life. To be at the foot of the cross and watch her beloved die, risking her own life to be there, meant that she too loved him to the very end, as he "loved his own who were in the world, he loved them to the end" (John 13:1).

"Going back to the beginning" meant understanding the spirituality of Mary Magdalene and the life she shared with Jesus as a woman who loved with her whole heart. As given to us in the Gospels of Mary and Philip, Mary Magdalene was more than a woman healed by Jesus; she also was a woman who understood the teachings of Jesus and the spiritual path of transformation. According to the *Gospel of Philip,* Mary Magdalene was Jesus' *spiritual companion.*

Over time, even this perspective expanded. I began to discover that there are different layers of meaning in the revelation given to me to "return to the beginning." I began to feel that there was still more to the story, and going back into the story led me to diving deeper into the ancient spiritual traditions of Jesus' time and even before his time, wondering what he may have encountered in the sojourn between age 12 and his reappearance in the New Testament Scriptures at age 30.

Interestingly, what we know is that the Silk Road, the trade routes from the west to the East, passed through the town of Capernaum on the Sea of Galilee where Jesus walked, taught, and preached. Capernaum was strategically positioned on the crossroads of the regions' major highways, on the route from Jerusalem to Damascus, making it an important center of commerce. Trade routes were more than centers of goods and raw materials for trade; they were also the communications highways of the ancient world. New inventions, religious beliefs, artistic styles, languages, and social customs were also exchanged and transmitted by people conducting business along the routes. Could it be that transporters of spices coming from India could have brought teachings of their sciences with them, sparking a curiosity in Jesus? Could Jesus himself have sojourned along the Silk Road trade routes as a teenager or young adult with an adventurous spirit, seeking knowledge and cultural experiences, and perhaps even spiritual experiences?

As I explored "going back to the beginning," I discovered a perspective on Jesus' teachings based on the deeply spiritual writings of Paramahansa Yogananda, the great Indian yogi who brought yoga to the west. This led me to the discovery by Nicolas Notovitch in the late 1800s of the ancient texts of Jesus's sojourn in India. This seemed unthinkable—but I thought to myself, "Why not? Can't I at least explore this thread?"

Notovitch tells the story of his encounter with monks in northern India and Nepal in the 1880s that spoke of a Saint Issa from Israel "in whom was manifest the soul of the universe."[66] According to Notovitch, the monks believed there were ancient manuscripts that told of a "perfect Being, living about two thousand years ago, who incarnated himself to enlighten humanity on the life beyond the grave and, by his own example, to bring back men to the true way and into the path that might best lead them to original moral purity."[67] The manuscripts say that Issa went back to Israel, and later they found out that he had been assassinated.

Interestingly, from our Christian Scriptures, we know nothing about the life of Jesus from the time he was age 12 to the beginning of his ministry when he was 30. Could it be that this very holy man named Issa truly was Jesus, traveling all through India and in Nepal and Tibet, learning from the masters, and *integrating the ancient tradition of yoga and meditation* into his life? Could it be that Jesus integrated yogic practices into his life for interior transformation before he went back to do the work God had given him to do? Could it be possible that ancient yogic practices helped Jesus to remember—and rediscover in a deeper way—who he was and his life purpose? Whether or not you believe in this possibility—that the bridge between yogic practices and Christianity could have been built by Jesus himself—is not the point: the bridge is still relevant and deeply transformational for pilgrims on the journey of spiritual realization, especially those who engage the spiritual practices of yoga and meditation.

Yogananda also affirms that Swami Abhedananda travelled in 1922 to the Himis Monastery and confirmed the "salient details about Issa published in Notovitch's book."[68] The yogis of today also speak of the ancient teachings about Jesus. Robert Boustany, master yogi, spiritual teacher and one of my trusted yoga teachers, has trained under Himalayan yogi masters who continue the ancient teachings. Robert graciously shared with me the teachings of these Himalayan yogi masters who say that Jesus is the LORD of the yogis, LORD of the cosmos. They call him *Super Mani*, the One who symbolizes the method of great compassion and love. How interesting that the yogic tradition has known of Jesus throughout the millennia and respected and revered him as LORD. I wonder why this teaching is not more widely known. For those who call Jesus the Christ, this teaching is affirming; for Christians who practice yoga and meditation as spiritual disciplines, it is compelling and powerful.

The Christian Scriptures pick up when Jesus is about age 30. The Gospels tell us, especially the *Gospel of Mark*, that Jesus often went up to the mountain to pray alone. He went into deep prayer, deep union with God. *Jesus was a contemplative!* Jesus made time for quiet time to just *be* alone in God's presence and hear God's still, small voice. Jesus took great care to follow the words of the Psalmist: "Be still and know that I am God" (Psalm 46:10). It is not surprising that the recent discoveries of the "Eastern Canon" Gospels of Thomas, Philip and Mary reflect contemplative and spiritual practices of these early Christian communities. *The Gospel of Mary* reflects the spirituality of Mary Magdalene as a contemplative spirituality, where Mary transmits, as a spiritual teacher, all that the Master has taught her about ascension to the divine to be in union with God. In the *Gospel of Mary,* Mary spoke as an authority, as one to whom the Savior taught these contemplative practices. As Cynthia Bourgeault explains in her scholarly interpretation of the meaning of the *Gospel of Mary*, "The fruit of this (Mary's) work is not only psychological wholeness, but the capacity to see. Her clear heart is her intimate channel to the fullness beyond time."[69] Here we are invited to imagine the power of psychological and spiritual wholeness.

For early Christians who argued that Jesus was already fully human and fully divine—the Word since the beginning of time, at birth, and into the fullness of time—the spirituality of seeking union with the divine would be inconsistent, since he already was both fully human and fully divine. I often wonder about his young life, his spiritual awareness of himself and of God, and how his journey unfolded. I wonder if his own path was to discover or rediscover this union for himself, and then to teach this path of union so that others would come to know this very truth for themselves?

Even in his life, in his words and actions, we see Jesus as the one who points us to full union with God. He is one who is freed and completely liberated from all sin and any veils that would prevent him from seeing God and living in God, a soul completely free to *be* God walking on the earth. As we study the life of Christ and his teachings, we see an example of the fully manifested power of the human soul to love, to heal, to serve. We see in Jesus the full manifestation of the fruit of the Spirit as given to us by St. Paul in his letter to the people of Galatia: "But the fruit of the Spirit is love, joy, peace, patience, kindness, goodness, faithfulness" (Galatians 5:22). We see in Jesus in the *Gospel of Mary* a soul that has fully developed and liberated itself to the realm of silence.

Clearly, Jesus is the full representation of the path to wholeness. His life lived in pure thought and awareness of God's presence is seen through his teachings and his actions, through his willingness to passionately live, teach, and die for his truth, the truth of God's presence and love, and his path to discover the treasure of the kingdom of God both out there and also deeply within. For me, the very possibility that in his life he encountered the wholeness practices of yoga and meditation provides a deeply rich and more holistic picture of the life of Jesus, whom I follow and have given my life and ministry to share his teaching with others. It may mean that not only was Jesus a healer, and our Savior, but that he also knew the paths to physical, emotional, and spiritual healing that yogic practices offer, and he may have even taught them as well to his inner circle of disciples who were hungry for the interior, contemplative life.

I desire to follow Jesus and to try and live the way he lived, and when I make mistakes and hurt others and myself, I wish to make amends, to make it right as best as I can, and to be accountable to myself, others and God for my actions and their consequences. I do not always succeed, and if I am truthful with myself, this is a key component in my life's work—to heal the relationships with which I am unable to truly *be* love. I look to Jesus to show me how to live more compassionately toward myself and others, how to give of myself more freely to help others, and how to honor and love all and send out blessings. I look to Jesus to lead me back to God, to the deepest, intimate relationship with God possible, as I continue to grow in the life of the Spirit. And I welcome the spiritual practices of yoga and meditation to heal me and guide my walk with Jesus into the heart of God.

I want to be, as much as I am able, a full manifestation of a daughter of God, made in God's image. I want to reflect the presence of God within me and to walk in the awareness that God cannot be boxed in by words and images of either masculinity or femininity, or even religious language or traditions, but that God is all and in all. I want the clear heart of Mary Magdalene, who demonstrates the capacity to see with the eyes of her spiritual heart and to love with full abandon, being healed and made whole through her relationship with Jesus. I see her body and soul, and Jesus' body and soul, walking alongside each other on the roads of Palestine and the hills surrounding Jerusalem, on the cobblestone streets of Jerusalem, and ultimately their spirits meeting in the vast expanses beyond time and space. That is the story's "beginning" that I embrace with my whole heart.

## The Intersection of the Yoga Sutras of Patanjali with the Path of Jesus

The path of Jesus is exemplified through his birth, death, and resurrection. But there is more to Jesus, and it is his *life*. It is his spiritual life that teaches us how to live the Way in the everyday, ordinary days of our lives. We see so clearly in the Transfiguration the complete fullness of the glory of God: "And while he was praying, the appearance of his face changed, and his clothes became dazzling white" (Luke 9:29). Mystics and yogis know of holy people who become surrounded in white light; it is the highest spiritual realization of the yogic path.

Patanjali, in his *Sutras,* explained the path of Yoga that can ultimately bring one to the highest goal: to attain the highest *Samadhi,* or totally liberated state. One could argue that Jesus had reached this liberated state; how else could he allow himself to be subjected to authorities in such cruel ways and even then, love at all costs? For Patanjali, this liberation is not just a state for when we die, but a state for when we are alive, to be lived in the midst of our lives, in these bodies, in the world. Patanjali developed the

*Yoga Sutras* based on ancient yogic practices to provide a set of *sutras*, or laws, rules, methods and means to become fully human and fully integrated. This full integration can be likened to what it means to become Christ-like, as Jesus described: "You therefore must be perfect, as your heavenly Father is perfect" (Matthew 5:48). It helps me to think of perfection in the sense of wholeness and integration, and a pure heart unencumbered by attachments to what "should be" in our minds, and not what most people think of as a complete faultlessness, which in actuality would mean we are not human! What Jesus is saying appears to be a possibility for us humans that it *can* happen.

How, we might ask? In addition to the Christian Scriptures that so beautifully teach us right living, true worship, and compassion, *the Yoga Sutras* give us a picture, a model, of the soul's development and unfolding into its fullness, a system of spiritual progress toward a higher consciousness. Patanjali's *Sutras,* arising out of an entirely different culture and religious context from the Judeo-Christian context, surprisingly complement the teachings of Christ.

The exact history of Patanjali's *Sutras* is unknown. It is not known exactly when Sri Patanjali lived, or even if he was a single person or several persons using the same title. Estimates of the date of the *Sutras* range from 5,000 B.C. to 300 A.D, implying that the sciences were developed over time just as the sciences today are developed over time. Isn't it interesting how much more we know about medicine, the mind, and the body today than we did even a few decades ago? Or how much more we know about the planets and our universe today, with the Hubble Space Telescope launched in 1990, and astronomers, astronauts, and scientists mining and exploring our cosmos and star constellations for new knowledge? In the same way, can what we know and experience about God also grow and develop over time?

The *Sutras* are a collection of "threads" that probe the mysteries of the mind and consciousness, referring to a type of Yoga called "Raja Yoga," the mental science. The word *raja* means king in Sanskrit, and the expression Raja Yoga implies a complete mastery of the Self in life. To better understand the contributions of Patanjali's Sutras, Sri Swami Satchidananada offers their historical importance:

> "[Patanjali] did not 'invent' Raja Yoga; what he offered humankind was a systematization of it and compiled the already existing ideas and practices [that had been passed down through oral tradition]. Since the time of his writing, Patanjali has been considered the 'Father of Yoga' and his *Sutras* are the basis for the various types of meditation and Yoga which flourish today in their myriad forms."[70]

Students of yoga philosophy learn in the *Sutras* how to be fully human. As the world continues to separate "us" and "them," the practice of becoming fully human is a way forward to bringing compassion into the world, for as one becomes fully human, it becomes difficult to ignore the fact that your neighbor is also human and part of the same inter-related systems of science and nature in which we all live.

B.K.S. Iyengar, one of the foremost teachers of yoga in our time, said that Patanjali's explanation of ways to control the mind are not referred to as Raja Yoga but as Ashtanga Yoga or the eight stages (limbs of Yoga)."[71] In contrast to the mental science of Raja Yoga, Hatha Yoga is the physical discipline of *asanas* and *pranayama* (breath control to influence the flow of *prana* or life force). Many people seeking yoga for medical benefits and overall good health will attend classes that offer physical yoga, or Hatha Yoga. Hatha Yoga is, however, more than physical yoga.

Iyengar explains: "The *Hatha Yoga Pradipika* of Swami Swatmarama, the classic Sanskrit manual on Hatha Yoga, deals solely with physical discipline. *The Yoga Sutras* of Patanjali deal with spiritual discipline, and these two Yogas [Raja and Hatha] complement each other on the path to freedom and Liberation."[72] In the 20th century, the physical postures, or *asanas*, have become popular and are simply called "yoga," although this is only one of the eight branches of yoga as outlined in the *Sutras*.

Patanjali's Yoga *Sutras*, or eight limbs of yoga, provide a framework for the quest of the soul. As I listen to my own heart, I hear a deep longing for God, and am grateful for discovering the yogic path to God that acknowledges my body, my actual physical presence in this life, and guides me in ways to calm the mind for ease in opening to the presence of God. It is helpful to have an understanding of the eight limbs of yoga to listen for the "sympathetic strings" and how Yoga can inform the Christian path to deeper faith development and union with the divine.

For comparative illustration, the following table demonstrates the sympathetic strings of Patanjali's eight limbs of yoga and the Christian path:

| Patanjali's Eight Limbs of Yoga | Sympathetic Strings | The Christian Path |
|---|---|---|
| **Yamas** - five rules of moral code:<br><br>*ahimsa* (non-violence)<br><br>*satya* (honesty, truthfulness)<br><br>*asteya* (non-stealing)<br><br>*brahmacharya* (wise and moderate use of energy, including sexual energy)<br><br>*aparigraha* (non-possessiveness, not being covetous or greedy, not accumulating beyond what is essential) | Moral restraints for relating to others that allow us to be at peace with ourselves, our family, our community, and with God<br><br>"You shall not" | **Deuteronomy 12:**<br>You shall not murder. *(ahimsa)*<br><br>Neither shall you commit adultery. *(satya, asteya)*<br><br>Neither shall you steal. *(asteya)*<br><br>Neither shall you bear false witness against your neighbor. *(satya)*<br><br>Neither shall you covet anything that belongs to your neighbor. *(aparigraha)* |

| Patanjali's Eight Limbs of Yoga | Sympathetic Strings | The Christian Path |
|---|---|---|
| The **Niyamas** are five rules of personal behavior:<br><br>*saucha* (purity)<br><br>*santosha* (contentment)<br><br>*tapas* (discipline or austerity)<br><br>*svadhyaya* (studies of the sacred texts)<br><br>*Ishvara Pranidhana* (constant awareness of and surrender to divine presence) | Observances for relating to ourselves that allow us to be at peace with ourselves, our family, our community, and with God<br><br>"You shall" | "Be perfect, therefore, as your heavenly Father is perfect." **(Matthew 5:48)** *(saucha)*<br><br>Jesus said, "Therefore do not worry, saying, 'What will we eat?' or 'What will we drink?' or 'What will we wear?'" **(Matthew 6:31)** *(santosha)*<br><br>After three days they found him in the temple, sitting among the teachers, listening to them and asking them questions. **(Luke 2:46)** *(svadhyaya)*<br><br>"Pray without ceasing." **(1 Thessalonians 5:17)** *(Ishvara Pranidhana)* |

| Patanjali's Eight Limbs of Yoga | Sympathetic Strings | The Christian Path |
|---|---|---|
| *Asana* refers to yoga postures and physical yoga that keep the body strong, flexible, relaxed and at ease.<br><br>Included in Patanjali's initial practice as the preparation of the body to sit still for meditation. | Preparation of the body for meditation. | Present your bodies as a living sacrifice, holy and acceptable to God, which is your spiritual worship. **(Romans 12:1)** |
| *Pranayama* are yoga breathing techniques designed to control and regulate *prana*, the breath, the energetic life-force. | The different methods of breathing can build heat, reduce anxiety, raise and control energy, and raise conscious awareness of being and of God's presence. | Then the Lord God formed man from the dust of the ground, and breathed into his nostrils the breath of life; and the man became a living being. **(Genesis 2:7)**<br><br>Jesus said, "Someone touched me; for I noticed that power had gone out from me." **(Luke 8:46)** |

| Patanjali's Eight Limbs of Yoga | Sympathetic Strings | The Christian Path |
|---|---|---|
| *Pratyahara* is the drawing of one's attention toward silence with internal stabilization of the senses. | Contemplative practices to rest in God, withdraw from the senses, go inward, and develop inward energy flow. | Jesus went to a mountain to pray. **(Luke 6:12)** |
| *Dharana* is meditation, concentration of the mind, to cultivate inner perceptual awareness. | Another term for meditation | In Christian language, we call this Meditation, Centering Prayer, or Contemplative Prayer |
| *Dhyana* is absorption through meditation, an expansion that sustains awareness under all conditions. | Higher spiritual consciousness as a result of meditation and moving beyond the mind where energy flows continually in the spiritual heart. | And he was transfigured before them, and his face shone like the sun, and his clothes became dazzling white. **(Matthew 17:2)** |

| Patanjali's Eight Limbs of Yoga | Sympathetic Strings | The Christian Path |
|---|---|---|
| *Samadhi* is integration, enlightenment, union with the divine, the return of the mind into original silence. | Pure devotion, deep realization and inner union, and pure, unobstructed energy flow in the spiritual heart. | Jesus said, "The glory that you have given me I have given them, so that they may be one, as we are one." **(John 17:22)**<br><br>Yeshua answered, "It is only at your source that you will find your destiny. Blessed are those who come to stand in their place of origination, for it is there that they will know their end—never tasting death." **(*Gospel of Thomas*, Logion 18)** |

As you can see, the Yoga *Sutras* of Patanjali in fact are resonant with the Ten Commandments as illustrated above; they are not in contradiction to the laws of the Judeo-Christian faith and they also resonate with the Christian path and the New Testament Christian Scriptures in interesting ways. The *Sutras* simply add tools, methods, and techniques for the spiritual aspirant, and the follower of Christ, to achieve greater clarity on the path to awakening to God's presence. By offering physical postures, breathing techniques, control of the senses, meditation, and other methods to discover the presence of God, the *Sutras* provide a path for the "how" that I, and many, seek.

When we set out on a vacation, we have a destination in mind. We use maps, or satellite directions, to help us navigate toward our destination. We wouldn't think of leaving our familiar surroundings without any directions. Yet for some, in the Christian spiritual life, a complete structure or framework for experiencing God is lacking. We have built intellectual methods and systematic theology for understanding God, yet people are seeking to discover God for themselves through their *own* spiritual experience. The "how to" of the *Yoga Sutras* can be useful by providing a set of experiential tools that help one to discover the presence of God's energy or Spirit within one's self. These can be helpful additions to the spiritual practices of journaling, devotional prayers, study, *Lectio Divina* or sacred reading, prayer beads, and walking the labyrinth. Practicing yoga, breath work, and meditation are complementary spiritual practices to traditional forms of intercessory and devotional Christian prayer. *Alongside* prayer, they offer greater choices for self-realization. *As* prayer, they open us to the personal experience of oneness with God.

People often ask me, "How should I pray?" I point the aspirant to the Lord's Prayer (Matthew 6:9-13) and to the wise instruction of Jesus when he said to his disciples: "But whenever you pray, go into your room and shut the door and pray to your Father who is in secret; and your Father who sees in secret will reward you." The silent prayer of the heart—meditation and contemplative prayer—is a way to experience union with God. Often people also ask me, "How do I really know if it is God talking to me?" When we listen to God in the silence, it is up to each of us to discern if the voice we hear is God's voice or our own, and to respond gladly when we hear God speaking, responding as Samuel did: "Speak, for your servant is listening" (1 Samuel 3:10b).

As a Christian, I have become curious about the methods prescribed in the yogic science of the mind as a means to engage the soul's quest for God. Every day, I start with twenty minutes of silent Christian meditation to come physically, emotionally, mentally and spiritually into God's presence, and I practice at least ten minutes of yoga to ground me (twenty to forty minutes is much better, but ten minutes will do if I'm in a hurry). These are the times when Patanjali's *Sutras* resonate with me most clearly; these are the moments when the "sympathetic strings" play a melodic vibration in my soul to revive me, to bring me back to a state of groundedness, dropping into the greater power of God. I am again integrated and experiencing a state of knowing and loving God personally and intimately. My heart comes home and I am grounded, open, and ready to receive what the day will bring, with prayers for God to show me who and how I should serve, and prayers for the grace to follow the Spirit's leading and remain open to the flow of the Spirit as life unfolds. When I begin my day in this groundedness, and am able to continue staying in my heart space throughout my day, my life seems to flow effortlessly, with sacredness to it all. My actions, my words, my movements become a living prayer.

Staying grounded with an open heart is resonant with Jesus' simple commandment that summed up all the commandments and laws of the Hebrew Scriptures: *the greatest commandment of all is to love God with all that you are* [my interpretation]. He went beyond that one greatest commandment, and added a second: *to treat others, and yourself, with the deepest love and respect* [my interpretation]. In Jesus' words,

> "'You shall love the Lord your God with all your heart, and with all your soul, and with all your mind.' This is the greatest and first commandment. And a second is like it: 'You shall love your neighbor as yourself'" (Matthew 22:37-39).

It's the "as yourself" part that trips up most of us. Many struggle with loving themselves, with understanding how much God loves them. Even as an Episcopal Priest, I confess that I want to love myself, I want to feel valued and worthy, I want to feel "good enough," and yet sometimes I don't. Others, too, admit they often feel the same way. We know in our heads that God loves us, but really believing it, and getting it into our hearts in a lasting way is difficult and challenging, and often feels nearly impossible.

This is where the Yoga *Sutras* can be useful. They provide a roadmap for me to quiet my mind when it tells me I'm not good enough. Engaging in *asana, pranayama,* and *dharana* help me understand how my body can be a vehicle for discovering God. They give me tools for breathing, meditating, and moving my body that helps me discover the joys of being human. The *Sutras* are complementary to my Christian faith and give me tools I wouldn't otherwise have. I am grateful to the ancient Indian sages and to Patanjali for giving the world a method, a set of "threads" that can be woven together, to help me in my quest for God and in my quest for finding peace within. Now, gratefully, we have a pathway, a set of tools in the *Sutras* to help us discover the healing and wholeness necessary for moving toward the higher Self, the True Self made in the *Imago Dei*, the image of God. The *Sutras* are "sympathetic strings" to Christian ethics, and to the Christian spiritual life, taking me deeper in my outward and inward journeys to experiencing wholeness and union with God, waking up to my true nature in God.

## Fulfilling Life's Purpose is Returning to Soul

When I was hearing my call to ordained ministry, I talked to everyone I could who was in ministry. I read every book on vocation and discernment I could find. My quest for knowledge led me to discover as much as I could about the path I would be entering. The heart knew, but my mind so very much wanted to be in control.

People ask me, "How did you hear your call to ministry? Why did you decide to leave corporate America to be a priest?" It was a long hard road of discernment for me, because I wanted to be "in charge" of my life. I had worked hard to earn my education in Business Statistics and my Masters of Business Administration. I had worked hard in project management and human resources leadership to have a fulfilling and rewarding career. But God just kept calling me to pray. When I learned of the lives of the saints of the church, I better understood the depth of what it means to follow Jesus with your whole life. I was restless, and I couldn't sleep. My answer to the question, "How did you know?" is simple: I couldn't sleep, deeply sleep, for two years. A kind priest and friend, The Reverend Dr. Mark Crawford, graciously led me through the Ignatian Exercises for discernment of my call, patiently listening to my inner struggle. Grateful for his compassion, I finally was able to say out loud what my heart knew: "Yes, I am called to go to seminary, and to follow God's leading. Actually, there is no other way, if I want peace."

When we open our heart to hear God's calling for our life's purpose, we may experience internal conflict and turmoil, because our old paradigm may be shaken to its core. All that we thought we wanted and worked for could shift. Yet I am convinced God uses all that we did before we hear the calling as we embrace a new way of life. And we also may experience external conflict as the people we love and who support us may not understand, they may not support us to go down a new path, or the changes may drastically impact their lives too in unexpected ways.

We may decide to not follow our true calling, and even then, the calling doesn't go away. It takes courage and creativity to step into the unknown. Not everyone wants to go there. As my yoga teacher Robert Boustany says, "This is your life." We are each responsible for creating our path and living life to the fullest.

The heart knows. You get to a point where your heart just knows. That is God speaking in the depths of your soul. Clarity, clear awareness, and conviction become seated deep within. As Joan Chittister says in her *Rule of Benedict* Commentary, "The will of God for us is what remains of a situation after we try without stint and pray without ceasing to change it."[73] Finally surrendering to that which is, and saying yes, you begin to feel free and open. A new sense of well-being sets in when you know you are on your path. This is a transformational time: a little, or deeply unsettling, but oh so exciting!

Living in God, for God and with God is simply the best way to live a full and rewarding life. Spiritual practices aid in spiritual progress for listening to the divine calling for your unique life. Whatever spiritual practice opens you to the divine is worth exploring. Lauren Artress said, "Opening to the sacred is a profound, life-changing process. It frees enormous energy that needs to be channeled back out into the world in service."[74]

In spiritual direction, I seek to help others find the answers to these questions: "What is it that God is calling you to do? How can you align your life with God's will?" This is about attending to your passions that God has placed on your heart, and using your talents, skills and gifts to live into your passionate desire to make the world a better place, to usher in God's kingdom "on earth as it is in heaven."

God's will for our lives is always grounded in love, for God, for our neighbors, for ourselves. It always goes beyond us, and yet it begins by knowing yourself. One of my favorite sayings of Frederick Buechner is given in his book *Wishful Thinking,* which beautifully describes God's will for your life, your vocation—or perhaps just the next chapter of your life:

> "The place God calls you to is the place where your deep gladness and the world's deep hunger meet."

In selfless service, we find God's peace. We discover our true essence when we meet another's needs and touch their hearts. So many want to know how to discern their life's purpose. I teach spiritual gifts classes in the church that help people to see where God has gifted them that may offer insight into passions and personality traits that further clarify their talents and possible direction. Some people are disconnected from their innermost feelings and intuition, and most people are disconnected from their bodies and what their bodies are teaching them. Therefore, they do not recognize their own feedback system, and do not understand the language of their inner voice, the interior language of the body-mind-soul-spirit. We can listen for what feels right inside, and for what feels discordant with our inner knowing. Listening to our interior language gets us closer and closer to wholeness and our inner truth that God beckons us to hear.

It is when we go back to the beginning, sitting in the silence of the cave of the heart, that we hear the gentle nudging and longings of the soul. As I leaned in, closer and closer, I heard God whispering to me..."Go back to the beginning...remember who you are."

## ~7~

# Awakening –
## *Healing and Inner Knowing*

Our purpose becomes not to try to understand God,
but to understand what it means to be human, or as
much as we can within the constraints of this time-
bound ego and body we have been given.

*–J. Pittman McGehee and Damon J. Thomas*[75]

### The Body Awakens to the Power to Heal Itself

Many people practice yoga for its health benefits. Yoga is a
fitness craze, being taught in fitness and yoga studios and clubs in
the US and around the world—sometimes in classes as large as
70 or 100 people moving in rhythm, focusing on firm abs, arm
and leg strength, and sweaty success. The "Just Do It" motto
underlies our cultural workout regimens and motivates us to do
more and do it now!

A healthy body contributes to a healthy mind. A healthy
body leads to vitality and more enjoyment of life. Life is a gift. I
love that well-known quote from Mary Oliver: "Tell me, what
is it you plan to do with your one wild and precious life?" The
practice of yoga takes us deeper into that amazing question as we
explore layers of ourselves on the mat and in meditation. Yoga
practitioners often say they wake up one day and face a choice
on how they will live their lives—either on the same path they
have set for themselves (and often feel stuck in) or exploring new

opportunities that the practice of yoga gives them the courage to discover. We don't have to apologize for wanting to live into our wild and precious lives, but choosing the exploration often comes with self-doubt, fear, and anxiety.

The physical healing that comes with the practice of yoga *asanas* cannot be denied. The healing isn't a guarantee, but it is so inspiring to hear the many stories of people suffering from injuries, lower back pain, knee pain, post-traumatic stress disorder, fear, doubt, anxiety, and even depression, who have experienced some healing from practicing yoga.

I suffer from mild depression periodically in my life. Depression can be situational, and it can also be a genetic disposition that impacts the chemical balances in the brain. As a teenager, I can now see that my adventurous self also self-medicated my feelings of sadness and intermittent mild depression with alcohol and recreational drug use. That was the only way I knew to deal with the pain and confusion without having to ask for help. I lived by the motto, "If it feels good, do it!" As I look back in reflection, (and not excusing my behavior), I realize I really just wanted, and needed, to feel better.

When I discovered meditation, the impact was profound. My brain began to heal and actually allowed me to feel what I was feeling. My thoughts of "I can't do this," became instead, "I will be okay." A deep sense of God's abiding love for me began to permeate my existence that over time began to displace the depression. I began to awaken to a new perspective to "seeing" myself with God's eyes. When the depression began to settle in again, I also discovered a way to pray that became a meditative mantra for me. This mantra is from Psalm 23, and it is simple, repeating one phrase over and over and over in prayer to God: "Restore my soul. Restore my soul." I was heeding the advice of St. Paul, who says, "Pray ceaselessly." I repeated that mantra as often and as long as necessary, sometimes as long as twelve days straight before the sadness would mercifully lift. The meditation practice took me deeper into a restorative mode. And then I discovered that in my yoga practice *asanas*, too, were taking me deeper into restoration and healing.

The yoga practice of *asanas* helped me to move the body in a way that cleared stuck energy and released many of the feelings of sadness. In a particular pose, I would feel tears welling up as the release was occurring. The feelings coming up and though me, and finally being released, are an essential part of the human experience. Fully being human means feeling everything, and not avoiding it, denying it, and self-medicating it. The practice of yoga brought me deep healing for my depression as the situations and feelings associated with them were released. Deep-seated emotions of abandonment, lack of trust, betrayal, and anger—whatever the root cause of emotional pain—yoga will help it to come up and out of the body, freeing the body to heal on deeper and deeper levels.

Like many people, I suffer from lower back pain. Even though I was taught to have good posture, I often sit and stand in ways that exacerbate lower back pain (slouching, standing with hip to one side). Now that I practice yoga on my mat every day, I am more aware of my posture and I don't experience the lower back pain as often. Freedom from pain creates a renewed enthusiasm for life. I can do more. I have more positive feelings. Robert Boustany, founder of the Pralaya Yoga system, taught me a standing posture that has made all the difference when I'm standing for an extended period, such as standing in line, or standing to celebrate the Eucharist. With feet hip distance apart, engage the thighs and pull them away from each other, toward the outer line of the legs. You will feel a pull across the lower back and the sacrum. As the sacrum widens along the lower back, a sense of well-being arises when the pain releases. A simple shift in the standing posture can make all the difference in how you feel.

As keepers of these bodies, we have the choice to engage in practices that make our bodies feel well. We can affect our pain to a certain extent. We can affect our energy levels through movement, breathing, and good nutrition. When we are in pain in an area of our body, we can give it our full attention, focusing intentionally with undivided attention on the area experiencing the pain, breathing into it, having compassion for it, and loving it back to good health. When we add prayer for healing, we deepen the healing by invoking the power of the Holy Spirit, connecting the power and energy of God's Holy Spirit with ourselves. The energies of God joined with a personal intention to heal and improve health are a powerful combination.

In Scripture, we find several passages where Jesus addresses our intention to choose to engage life:

> James and John, the sons of Zebedee, came forward to him and said to him, 'Teacher, we want you to do for us whatever we ask of you.' And he said to them, 'What is it you want me to do for you?' (Mark 10:35–36)

> They came to Jericho. As he and his disciples and a large crowd were leaving Jericho, Bartimaeus son of Timaeus, a blind beggar, was sitting by the roadside. When he heard that it was Jesus of Nazareth, he began to shout out and say, 'Jesus, Son of David, have mercy on me!' Many sternly ordered him to be quiet, but he cried out even more loudly, 'Son of David, have mercy on me!' Jesus stood still and said, 'Call him here.' And they called the blind man, saying to him, 'Take heart; get up, he is calling you.' So throwing off his cloak, he sprang up and came to Jesus. Then Jesus said to him, 'What do you want me to do for you?' The blind man said to him, 'My teacher, let me see again.' Jesus said to him, 'Go; your faith has made you well.' Immediately he regained his sight and followed him on the way. (Mark 10:46–52).

I have experienced a healing of my heart by asking Jesus for what I need in prayer. Engaging in deep prayer for healing, asking for what I needed, and sitting in the silence and stillness of meditation brought me a deep healing and sense of peace; as we say in faith: the peace that passes all understanding, the peace of Christ, the peace that only God can give. One particular and profound healing happened in a beautiful setting, in Tuscany, Italy. I was on retreat at Monte Oliveto Monastery with the World Community for Christian Meditation, led by Father Laurence Freeman. Benedictine Oblates, an order of lay people who have taken monastic vows and who choose to live outside of the monastery and in the world, were gathered from around the world for a week-long silent retreat with Fr. Laurence Freeman and to experience the depths of silent meditation in that beautiful, sacred setting.

One afternoon, after our silent lunch, we had a long break to write, study, pray, sleep, shower, or walk on the grounds and experience the countryside. Free time gives the soul space to breathe and to listen to God. I went for a walk under the tall trees amidst the natural gardens. I found an old, short, stone wall under the trees and decided this was a perfect spot to sit and write as I opened my heart for God's guidance. I was in the early discernment process to leave my position at the university and enter seminary for full-time ministry. I was afraid and yet excited, hesitant and yet willing. My heart was conflicted as I spiritually stood between both ways of life, not yet knowing clearly how and when my path would bring me into a vocation to serve God in the church. Over the years, people have visited me with this same conflicting sense of call. It's a difficult place to be, and is only relieved by God's grace, and in God's time, when the heart fully surrenders to what God is saying to it.

I wrote in my journal, words flowing easily and quickly as I poured my heart out with questions of why, what, when, and how. I felt the call, I felt the yearning, and yet it was not in my control, and it was causing my life to feel out of control. I was writing this prayer, "Help me, God, please, and now! Show me and lead me out of my discomfort, open or close doors as you need for my life. Your will be done. Come, Lord Jesus, come." Finally, I put down my pen and begin to sit in the silence, feeling the warmth of the sun on my face and on my arms. Repeating my sacred mantra silently, in rhythm with my breath, "Ma-ra-na-tha" ("Come Lord" in Aramaic), I began to feel a sense of rest, peace, a quiet calm moving through my body. Warmth began to center into my chest, and I saw a vision of my heart opening, and warm, pure light energy was being poured into it. The warm, white-yellow light filled my heart completely, and then it gently sealed up. I knew in that moment I had received what I needed. My heart had been made whole. All the wounds from my life were healed with the pure light. My heart was light and no longer heavy. I knew my heart had been made ready for the journey ahead, wherever God would lead.

## The Mind and Soul as Integral Components of the Healing Process

As I spoke of earlier, yoga has helped me with a mild depression that has plagued me all of my life. On many days, even now, that nagging sense of meaningless pervades from the moment I awake in the morning. I pray once again for God to restore my soul, and then I sit for my daily twenty-minute silent Christian meditation practice as taught by the World Community for Christian Meditation. My mild depression sometimes still seems to hover over me with a numbing feeling of sadness that is unexplainable—it's just there. When I have been able to rise above it, to hover over myself, watching myself, I see sadness. Talking with other women, I have discovered that this is too is something many of us share—and in part, I believe, it is because we are sensitive to the collective sadness in our society. There are so many things to grieve over—crimes against our humanity, against our planet earth, against our children, against our bodies and our souls. This sadness is a collective sadness in our modern world and in our history, over the millennia, as we have seen women, men, and children suffer. My Self that "witnesses" this sadness knows that this feeling of sadness doesn't define me, and it doesn't define the totality of who I am or the message of abiding joy and hope that I feel called to share. So, even though I sometimes feel the sadness, I continue on anyway, doing what I am led to do, following the Spirit's leading, deeply connected to all of my emotions and to my heart space.

As an Episcopal priest and a spiritual director, I am intuitively and humbly aware of God's ever-present closeness, guidance, and movement in my life. My unfailing spiritual director has always been God, and thank goodness God also speaks loudly at times through real people. One spiritual director asked me so poignantly, "When have you known joy?" Her question was like a piercing arrow that went straight into my heart, and my body was unable to move. Holding back tears, the common theme of my life was exposed: sadness. A vulnerable place to be, for sure. This is a good question for all of us, and I invite you to reflect from your own heart space, "When have you known joy?" When you reflect on this question, where does it lead you, and how can it help you find your way into moving forward in your life?

I'm not a negative person. In fact, I am a hopeful person, so much that I have been accused of being an optimist! Even when there is no apparent or good reason to be optimistic, there it is anyway—unconscious and resilient optimism! My response to my accusers is that to view the glass as half full is that much sweeter when one has known the depths of sadness. For me, life is a deeply faithful choice to live fully, completely, and vulnerably, even when sadness tries to creep in, from life experience and circumstances, or from depression. In the *Gospel of John*, we are given words that encourage those stumbling around in the darkness:

> "The light shines in the darkness, and the darkness
> did not overcome it" (John 1:5).

That is my life story, an interplay of dark and light. Faith in God, personal and spiritual encounters with Jesus, the practice of gratitude for everything—even challenges—and the faithful and disciplined practice of yoga and meditation have transformed me and given me an abiding sense of hope. My depression over time has slowed in frequency and lasts only a short while; sometimes only minutes if I am able to get on yoga mat and work it out. Yoga helps me focus my rational mind in the present and allows my body and mind to heal itself. Meditation brings me back to my heart space where I find God in the silence, and I discover once again I am okay. I am Beloved. I am Spirit.

## The Human Energy System

Human beings are more than just physical, emotional, psychological, social, and spiritual beings. We are also beings of energy. In the physical body, we have two types of energy that supply the organs: *prana,* Sanskrit for "life force" energy, and the mind or consciousness. Swami Satyananda Saraswati describes how the body supplies energy:

> Modern physiology describes two types of nervous systems—the sympathetic and the parasympathetic, and these two nervous systems are interconnected in each and every organ of the body. In the same way, every organ is supplied with the energy of *prana* and the energy of mind.

> In yoga, the concept of *prana* is very scientific. When we speak of *prana*, we do not mean the breath, air or oxygen. Precisely and scientifically speaking, *prana* means the original life force.[76]

The yogic practice of managing breath or life force is called *pranayama*. It is an essential component to managing the variations in the mind, or what is referred to in meditation as the "monkey mind" that swings from limb to limb, thought to thought, always restless, never still. Learning to manage the mind through controlling the *prana* or life force is the work of *Hatha Yoga*. The purpose of Hatha Yoga is also to align the body's skin, bones, and muscles and to open the body's energy channels and activate the body's energy centers through yoga *asanas*. The two syllables *ha* and *tha* symbolize the "Sun" and the "Moon" and correspond to the right and left energetic pathways in the body called the *pingala nadi* (pathway) and the *ida nadi*. These two currents correspond to the sympathetic and parasympathetic nervous systems, and through the practice of Hatha Yoga, balance, ease and tranquility can be achieved.

Our bodies are extensions of universal matter and energy, and just as in the universe, solar and lunar energies are also present in the body. In yogic practice, solar energies are present in the right pathway or *pingala,* and lunar energies are present in the left pathway or *ida*. There is an interesting correlation between the yogic energetic pathways and psychological archetypes as Carl Jung described them. Viewing them in a holistic way, we gain a deeper understanding of how yoga and psychological integration offer an integral approach toward holistic healing and wholeness. When the energies within are balanced and in harmony, a deeper sense of peace and stillness in the body and mind are achieved.

In Jung's archetypal energy framework, there are solar and lunar energies. Jung's masculine archetypal energy, as mentioned earlier, is *Logos,* symbolized as solar, heating energy, just as the sun provides bright light and heat. Jung's feminine archetypal energy, *Eros*, is represented as lunar, cooling energy, just as the moon provides soft light while the earth and all life force upon it cool down at night. In yoga, the right energetic pathway is the solar energy current—like that of Jung's masculine energy—and the left energetic pathway is the lunar energy current—like that of Jung's feminine energy. In their totality, these archetypes, as in the yogic system of *nadis* or energy channels, impact how we feel, think, behave, respond, react, and project ourselves out into the world around us. These energies are inclusive of the human as biological, psychological, social, and spiritual beings.

Yoga practices recognize and seek to manage the energy flows within. Yoga *asanas* help to balance the energies and to clear blockages in energy flow. *Pranayama* manages the movement of breath within the body and directs it to specific areas of the body. Practicing yoga *asanas* can help to bring healing and to balance the masculine and feminine energies—the heating and cooling energies in the body and the mind—even when one is unaware of the positive effects of the practice.

The body's energy centers are known in Yoga as the *chakra* system. The chakra system is the entryway to the human energy body that each and every one of us has. The word *chakra* is a Sanskrit word and translates as "wheel" or disk." Anodea Judith describes a *chakra* as a center of activity, a wheel of spinning energy in the body for "the reception, assimilation, and expression of life force energy....The *chakra* refers to a spinning sphere of bioenergetics activity emanating from the major nerve ganglia branching forth from the spinal column. There are seven of these wheels stacked in a column of energy that spans from the base of the spine to the top of the head....The seven major chakras correlate with basic states of consciousness."[77]

We can't see the chakra system, since it's made of energy: it's invisible, in the same way that radio waves are invisible. If we are willing to acknowledge its existence, however, and we balance and heal the chakra system, the energy of the universal consciousness can work through us. Similarly, when we practice the laying on of hands to help another person heal and we call or invoke the consciousness of Jesus (Christ Consciousness), his healing power or energy works through us to address the physical, subtle and energy bodies—and the soul—of the one we are praying for. The rational mind is an active player, but we have to remember to let go of it and "get out of the way" so that our soul and psyche can be a channel for God's Spirit to flow.

Anodea Judith, authority on the integration of chakras and therapeutic issues, describes the connectedness of the mind to the body:

> Consciousness comes through that elusive entity we call the mind. It is our inner understanding, our memory, our dreams, and beliefs. It organizes sensate information. When consciousness is detached from the body, it is wide and vague, dreamy and empty, but capable of great journeys. When it is connected to our body, then we have a dynamic energy flow throughout our entire being. In this way, the spiritual realm becomes *embodied*, making it tangible and effective. In effect, we have plugged in the system, just as we plug in our radio, so we can tune in to various frequencies. The chakras then become like channels, receiving and broadcasting at different frequencies.[78]

The chakra system originated over four thousand years ago in India. According to Judith, they were first "referred to in the ancient literature of the Vedas, the later Upanishads, the *Yoga Sutras of Patanjali,* and most thoroughly in the sixteenth century by an Indian yogi in a text called the *Sat-Chakra-Nirupana.*"[79]

The ancient *chakra* system predates modern, Western medicine, but interestingly enough, there is a connection: the caduceus. You may have seen it; it is the symbol of the medical profession. It is a staff with two serpents wrapped around it, and wings at the top of the staff. Ken Wilber, American philosopher and author, describes the symbol as it relates to the chakra system:

> The staff itself represents the central spinal column; where the serpents cross the staff represents the individual *chakras* moving up the spine from the lowest to the highest; and the two serpents themselves represent solar and lunar (or masculine and feminine) energies *at each of the chakras.*[80]

Many Westerners are skeptical of the chakra system because we cannot see the chakras, and Western medicine traditionally has not recognized the subtle energy system in the body, for the same reason. (But how we love our wireless Internet connectivity!) The irony is that we choose to acknowledge energy outside of us but not inside of our bodies! Acupuncturists understand Chinese meridian lines in the body; yogis understand energy channels (*nadis*)—we each have *72,000* of these subtle energy channels in our bodies—and vortexes (*chakras*); and Western athletes understand the concept of needing to maintain high levels of energy for the sport. These different viewpoints represent different ways of accessing the same life force, or *prana*, and recognize the importance and criticality for balancing the energy system for healing and well-being.

To better understand the science of the yogic chakras, Anodea Judith provides this helpful description:

> Chakras are not physical entities in and of themselves. Like feelings or ideas, they cannot be held like a physical object, yet they have a strong effect on the body as they express the embodiment

of spiritual energy on the physical plane. Chakra patterns are programmed deep in the core of the mind-body interface and have a strong relationship with our physical functioning. Just as the emotions can and do effect our breathing, heart rate, and metabolism, the activities in the various chakras influence our glandular processes, body shape, chronic physical ailments, thoughts, and behaviors. By using techniques such as yoga, breathing, bioenergetics, physical exercises, meditation, and visualization, we can, in turn, influence our chakras, our health, and our lives. This is one of the essential values of this system—that it maps onto both the body and the mind, and can be accessed through either.[81]

There are, in actuality, many chakras in the human energy body; for our purposes here, I will focus on the seven major chakras. Everyone has these seven major *chakras* within their human energy body, connecting to their physical body and to seven corresponding levels of consciousness. These energy centers are located along the spine, extending out the front and back of the body, and ascend from the base of the spine to the crown of the head. Each chakra has specific energetic qualities that correspond to levels of consciousness; each has a direct relationship with our ability to progress spiritually since learning about them encourages us to master their essence and eventually unite them into a single field of radiant energy:

Root or Base Chakra, *Muladhara*, relates to security and survival

Sacral Area Chakra, *Svadhisthana*, relates to physical movement, mobility, creativity, sensuality, sexuality, and emotions

Solar Plexus Chakra, *Manipura*, relates to power, will, confidence, self-esteem, and energy

Heart Chakra, *Anahata*, relates love, harmony, balance, compassion, relationship, devotion, and intimacy

Throat Chakra, *Vissudha*, relates to communication, self-expression, and finding one's voice

Third Eye Chakra, *Ajna*, relates to vision, clarity, imagination, psychic perception, intuition, and symbolic expression

Crown Chakra, *Sahasrara*, relates to understanding, consciousness, mystery, eternity, divinity

You may be wondering how chakras relate to the spiritual life of a Christian. Since they exist in every human being, regardless of religious tradition, culture, ethnicity, or any other way one can construct a category or division, chakras are a universal truth for *every* human being, just as the physical anatomy structure of bones, muscles, and organs are true for everyone. And the proper functioning and balance of chakras is necessary for the health and well-being of the individual and the collective, because what affects one affects all.

Our inner healing is necessary for the spiritual life to progress. We must invite healing on every level: physically, emotionally, spiritually, and energetically. A holistic approach to healing (and medicine) recognizes the inter-relatedness of energy and illness. I hear stories of how energy medicine is healing people. One friend has cleared deep-seated feelings of inferiority and self-worthlessness and now has a new outlook on life with hope and perseverance. Another dear friend with a diagnosis of chronic leukemia has worked diligently through prayer, meditation, and yoga to place her cancer in remission, with the aid of traditional chemotherapy. A holistic approach to healing that includes yoga, nutrition, and energy medicine is a growing body of medical and scientific knowledge that may indeed contribute to the evolution of the human body and human consciousness.

Our growing knowledge ultimately must lead us to the healing of the heart, that one may find inner spiritual knowing. The heart is where we find our purpose, from where we offer our love and receive it, from where our offering to the world comes forth. Mystics throughout the ages have known how to tap into the heart center. Yogis view the heart center as the seat of the soul, the organ of cosmic intuition or consciousness. Other traditions value living from the heart center, as illustrated by Carl Jung in his book, *Memories, Dreams, Reflections*, as he reflected on meeting with Pueblo Indians and their discussion of the white man:

> "'They say they think with their heads,' said the Indian, having just told Jung that they thought the white man was 'mad.' Jung inquired what else could one think with and the Indian said, 'We think Here,' indicating his heart. Jung said that in that moment he saw Western Civilisation anew."[82]

Opening to another's viewpoint may create a catalyst for change. The heart center is where the intersection of the lower and upper chakras occurs, and it is usually where the greatest clearing is needed. The heart center feeds the upper chakras, and as it clears and becomes pure, the third eye chakra opens to a greater intuition and awareness, and the crown chakra opens to a higher consciousness.

This purifying or clearing is like that of God's refining fire... where the wheat and the chaff will be separated and "the chaff burned with unquenchable fire" (Matthew 3:12). This refining includes ethical behavior but goes beyond it to the heart center. Yoga gives us tools that help us love God and love our neighbors as ourselves by giving us a structure for clearing the heart and the body through chakra clearings and moving stuck energy to make room for that breadth and depth of love to blossom. It is hard to love others without fully loving ourselves and healing old wounds, so if we're harboring resentment, anger, hurt, grief, or other negative emotion, our entire self is not able to fully clear and grow into the fully realized, loving human being God intends for us to be. As author Jim Marion says of how we feel when we are free of blocked emotions, "Our emotions once more have the spontaneity of a child's."[83]

When the chakras are cleared, and the emotional and physical blockages are released, an opening in the crown chakra allows for an energetic exchange with the universal energy field. When I feel my crown chakra open, I literally feel the shape of a chalice coming out of the crown of my head and opening outward beyond me. This chalice represents my own outpouring into the world, my own self-giving to what is beyond me, to the greater collective consciousness.

Beautifully, this chalice at my crown chakra is also a receptacle. It is the place where my True Self receives the love and light that is pouring out for me from the mystical Christ. The consciousness of this mystical Christ pours into my crown chakra and enters into my mind, where my intellect and ego reside, and I feel deeply loved. I feel the love of Christ enter my being and this Christ Consciousness permeates me. As this conscious energy moves down into my throat and heart chakras, my physical being softens and relaxes as I receive. My breath softens. I feel an unconditional love and light tingling in me, energizing the cells in my body and awakening my soul to a deep sense of belonging and groundedness. When I am in this state of sharing and receiving, I am fully aware of God's presence around me and within me and of my connection with all of creation. My focus, my intention, my willingness to live in this presence determines the depth and length of the experience and my ability to remain in this clear awareness of God's presence.

To my surprise, I discover that I am not the first person to make the connection with the chalice of Christ Consciousness. Yogananda describes how it is available to us all:

> As Jesus received and reflected through his purified consciousness the divine sonship of Christ Consciousness, so also every man, by yoga meditation, can clarify his mind and become a diamond-like mentality who will receive and reflect the light of God.

Yogananda goes on to describe how yoga connects us to the Holy Spirit, which he calls the Cosmic Vibration:

> The method of contacting this Cosmic Vibration, the Holy Ghost, is for the first time being spread worldwide by means of definite meditation techniques of the *Kriya Yoga* science. Through the blessing of communion with the Holy Ghost, the cup of human consciousness is expanded to receive the ocean of Christ Consciousness. The adept in the practice of the science of *Kriya Yoga* who consciously experiences the presence of the Holy Ghost Comforter and merges in the Son, or immanent Christ Consciousness, attains thereby realization of God the Father and entry into the infinite kingdom of God.[84]

Meditation practice is a method of following Jesus into oneness and union with God. Somewhere I read that oneness is not a belief, but a state of consciousness. The yogis have known it, and

I believe the Christian mystics have known it too, through prayer. For Christians, a yoga and meditation practice can be viewed as simply God's grace leading us to this same divine awareness.

## Awakening to the Movement of the Spirit

Have you ever experienced an uncanny sense that you have had the same experience before—*déjà vu*? Or met someone and it seems like you have known them all of your life? Or sensed something will happen and then it does? I often do, and I call it my inner knowing, my intuition. I have a strong sense of intuition, and I usually base my decisions and my actions on my sense of this inner knowing, more than relying exclusively on reasoning. If it doesn't feel right deep within, then I know it isn't right for me.

A calling is like that. A calling leads you forward, sometimes propelling you so much that it doesn't feel like you are in control at all. The hard part for most of us is that we want to be in control, all the time. But with a calling, you just *know* you are supposed to do this, to keep moving ahead, to stay congruent, even and most especially if it wasn't your idea in the first place! Your intuition leads you, with a strong sixth chakra (your third eye) that is tapping into the universal life force, the Holy Spirit, to guide you forward. It is the movement of spirit, the eternal Self, as wisdom, the teacher within.

People often ask me, "How do you know?" I have often wished it were so simple as a neon sign flashing in front of me, giving me exactly the instructions I need to follow. It usually isn't so obvious; in fact, it is subtle, like a slight wind blowing that barely brushes your skin. This subtlety lies deep within, but it's there. It settles in, it creates a subtle wind of movement of energy within. When you are following your vocation, the energy quickens and fire develops within to propel you forward.

Everything in your life seems to flow in the same direction, validating and affirming your path. St. Ignatius of Loyola of 15th century Spain called this feeling "Consolation." Likewise, when you are moving away from your calling, the energy feels different—it feels like it is creating a distance, a disconnect, from where you are supposed to be going and what are you supposed to be doing. Your heart feels a gap, a void, an uneasiness. St. Ignatius of Loyola called this feeling "Desolation." Listening to your inner compass as a guide to the Spirit leading you and moving you forward can give you great clarity. At the right time, you will know what you are to do.

Discernment is learning to pay attention to these subtleties, to hear God's still, small voice within. When we are moved to pray it is because God is prompting us to pray. God wishes us to listen closely and deeply to the voice within and the movements within. The inner intuitive voice that nudges us gently, repeatedly until we listen, is the voice of God, calling us to deeper healing and inner knowing.

One of the appointed readings of Scripture for Pentecost Sunday, the day the church celebrates the Holy Spirit descending upon the people and making them one, tells us, "All who are led by the Spirit of God are children of God" (Romans 8:14). Being led by the Spirit of God requires openness to being led— to listening and then following. We can't hear if we are talking! We can't be led if we are leading and forcing our way! If we are willing to pay attention to the energy, to God's Spirit within, we enter into the awareness of God's flow for our lives.

Awakening is coming to the awareness of the presence of God's Spirit within. Awakening can be instantaneous, such as for St. Paul on the road to Damascus, or it can be a process in which an awakening happens, and then continues over and over again. I prefer the understanding that it is a lifelong process, a soul continually growing in depth and spiritual maturity. I choose to be awakened every day by that very Spirit bearing witness with my spirit that I am God's child (Romans 8:14-17). I am fully alive, walking and breathing in the ordinariness of life with the awareness that the I AM of God is the same I AM in each of us.

This is what Jesus meant when he said, "The kingdom of God is within you" (Luke 17:21b). People are hungry to feel God in their souls, to experience God. The church historically hasn't taught that we can find God inside, but many of the saints of the church have known it. If we heard it from Jesus but didn't believe it, then hopefully one of the great teachers, such as Thomas Merton, Laurence Freeman, Thomas Keating, Ram Dass, Richard Rohr, Cynthia Bourgeault, or many others can help you to understand it enough that you believe you can actually experience it for yourself. Whatever it takes. The important thing is that you get it and are able to become a fully conscious human being living in Christ Consciousness.

My own process of awakening has unfolded many times in meditation and on my yoga mat. On my mat, as I open up the body, getting the winds of energy to flow through me, I gain a sense of freedom, openness, and receptivity. The Spirit of God bears witness within me, teaching me what I need to know that day, at that very moment. I get messages that sustain me throughout the day or week, exactly what I need to hear and know right now. I get grounded in who I am and in my relationship with God, with the Spirit leading me. I am strengthened to follow God's Spirit into new areas of learning, discovery and relationship.

When I read Scripture, my inner knowing is strengthened by the words and the wisdom. When I am on my yoga mat, my inner knowing is developed intuitively, in a way that deepens my groundedness to what is and what will be.

When I first began to practice yoga as part of my spiritual path, some Christians pushed back, telling me it was un-Christian, that it would bring in foreign gods into my life, and even that it was demonic. I could see fear on their faces, their hearts on fire for Jesus but with a protective coating preventing anything different from the interpretation of Biblical Scripture they knew from entering their mindset. That's understandable. We know what we know. The challenge for me, as I said before, was that I loved Jesus, but I also loved yoga. I was conflicted internally also, but my inner knowing was that I needed yoga; it fed me, and it actually helped me heal on deeper levels and grow spiritually. My own Christian faith grew stronger, as if the words of Jesus, "But blessed are your eyes, for they see, and your ears, for they hear" (Matthew 13:16) were more clear to me than ever before.

And yet, there *was* that gnawing feeling of guilt—the guilt of turning away from the traditional teachings of the faith of my heritage. Born into a Christian family in Texas of German heritage, my family's religion is important. The Bible is the backbone of our values and the Holy Spirit our guide. So entering into a yoga studio with an image of Buddha's peaceful face on the wall, or a sculpture of the dancing *Nataraja*, the depiction of the Hindu god Shiva as the cosmic dancer who performs his divine dance (it took me seven years to learn who the image was), seemed unfaithful, as if I had betrayed someone—my family, God, even myself.

At first, in yoga classes, I couldn't chant with the group, fearing that the Sanskrit words might be in conflict with my religious beliefs. Even to chant the most basic word "Aum," the sound of eternal creation, felt like a betrayal. And yet, eventually I did chant Aum, and it felt good. The throat vibrates as the sound of Aum leaves the body...and energy begins to awaken the senses. Still, internal thoughts nagged at me: can I really practice yoga and chant these words? Is it safe, or will it lead me to leave my tradition, the way they say marijuana leads to heavier drugs? How does my yoga relate to my faith? Is it wrong even though it feels right?

I remembered that when I attended the silent retreat at the motherhouse monastery for the Benedictine Oblates of the World Community for Christian Meditation outside of Siena,

Italy, the same trip that opened my heart healing experience, we had practiced yoga every morning. We started our day in this beautiful stone monastery built in the 15th century to the sound of the monastery bells ringing from the chapel bell tower, beckoning the monks to the chapel for Morning Prayer. Our group silently made our way to the "upper room" where we met for silent meditation, with only words spoken for the opening and closing readings, and the sounds of our bell chimes ringing to start and end the meditation. The early morning breeze gently blew over our faces as the sun began to rise while we sat in the stillness and the silence, listening for God to speak to our hearts. Enjoying the feeling of coming home, listening to the birds beginning to sing their morning songs, we were one body, one heart, in this sacred place.

After a silent breakfast of fresh farm eggs, fruit and granola, the invitation to a morning yoga practice beckoned most of us back to our gathering room for an hour with a handsome, young Italian man who led us in gentle yoga—heart and hip openers, just what we needed for a day filled with lectures by our teacher, Fr. Laurence Freeman, OSB, and meditation sits. Our beautiful yoga teacher led us in body movements that opened us, and his teaching was poetic and beautiful. It was a time of spiritual awakening for me—like waking up from spiritual amnesia—to remembering who I was and all I already knew. In other words, my yoga practice did not require that I give anything up from my Christian faith; rather, it completely added to my love for God and Christ.

I found comfort that my life instructor and gospel teacher, Fr. Laurence Freeman, included yoga in his retreat—giving us a balance of teachings that opened our hearts, minds, *and* bodies. It seemed so sacred, so perfect. Yoga mats, yoga blankets, meditation chimes, the Gospel. I clearly knew that I had glimpsed heaven on earth in this holy monastery in a holy country with holy people.

That's how the process of awakening to the movement of spirit, the divine spark within, starts: opening. Heart, body, mind and soul ready to receive. Remembering. Awareness. The soul knows: I am here. Now. Alive. Embodied. And it is good. All good.

## Awakening to Who We Already Are

We can look to Jesus for the words that give life: "In fact, the kingdom of God is within you" (Luke 17:21b). Most English translations of the Greek words in this passage, "ἐντὸς ὑμῶν", ("entos hymōn") use "in the midst of you" rather than "within you." Christians hang our beliefs on the translations of the Greek New Testament, and how important it is that the translations be accurate and that they reflect the meaning that Jesus wished to convey. I was surprised to learn that the Greek interlinear translates "ἐντὸς ὑμῶν" as "inside of you." Could the words, "in the midst of you," or "among you" have meant "inside of you," or did they strictly refer to something outside of your body and your soul? After all these centuries, I can only wonder what Christianity would look like had the church taught followers of Jesus that the kingdom of God is inside each of us, and not only Jesus, the Son of God. Perhaps as our teacher, he is like the Buddha. Let me explain what I mean.

In his book, *Old Path, White Clouds*, Thich Nhat Hanh tells the story of the Buddha. The Buddha taught:

> "'My teaching is not a dogma or a doctrine, but no doubt some people will take it as such.'" The Buddha goes on to say, 'I must state clearly that my teaching is a method to experience reality and not reality itself, just as a finger pointing at the moon is not the moon itself. A thinking person

makes use of the finger to see the moon. A person who only looks at the finger and mistakes it for the moon will never see the real moon.'"[85]

Could Jesus be pointing us to seeing that within *each* of us lies the very possibility of union with God and Christ Consciousness? Bede Griffiths, the late British-born Christian Benedictine monk and priest who became a yogi in South India, understood the fruit of the spiritual path as self-realization:

> There is a point where intuition, having passed through the realms of darkness and of twilight into the Sun, now passes beyond. It carries with it all the deep experience of the body and the blood, and all that the emotions and the imagination have impressed upon it, and now passing beyond images and thoughts, it 'returns upon itself' in a pure act of self-reflection, of self-knowledge. This is the experience of the mystic, who, set free from all the limitations both of body and soul, enters into the pure joy of the spirit. The spirit is the culminating point of body and of soul, where the individual person transcends himself and awakens to the eternal ground of his being.[86]

Spiritual practices bring us deeper on the path to awakening to God. The church teaches spiritual practices, and the church brings us into the mystery of what these practices point to. Why not incorporate the spiritual practices of self-realization yoga in our religious lives to enrich and deepen our inner knowing? I doubt it is by coincidence that God's Holy Spirit has brought these spiritual practices to the West:

"Jesus said, 'The wind blows where it chooses, and you hear the sound of it, but you do not know where it comes from or where it goes. So it is with everyone who is born of the Spirit'" (John 3:8).

What more can we learn from these Eastern yogic practices? As I study and engage in the practice of yoga, illumined by Jesus' teachings in the *Gospels of Thomas* and *Mary*, my own faith in Jesus deepens. As a rabbi, teacher, healer, and spiritual master, his teachings are indeed congruent with the path of awakening. How does our faith walk change if we see that awakening to Christ Consciousness is where Jesus was ultimately trying to lead us?

# ～ 8 ～

# Embodied Spirituality –
## *Incarnation*

It is not about becoming spiritual beings nearly as much as about becoming human beings. The biblical revelation is saying that we are already spiritual beings; we just don't know it yet.

*—Richard Rohr*[87]

## In the Beginning

We come into the world as pure miracle, so innocent, so dependent upon another human being to take care of us, to give us what we need to survive and to feel nurtured, loved, and cared for. If we were blessed with a loving family, all we had to do was move our mouths in sucking gesture or a gentle smile, and parents and grandparents squealed with delight. When we cooed with our lips and our voices, adults responded with excitement. Parents and grandparents smiled and giggled with every sound, every potential word that we uttered. "Mmmmmm," that gentle humming sound, making bubbles with our mouths, sounding out the gentle OM that comes as naturally and instinctively as a bird learns to flap her wings to fly.

We hung out on our backs in happy baby pose, exploring what it feels like to stretch our legs overhead, to rock from side to side with legs suspended in the air, to hold our toes and pull and tug, to grab our feet and pull them down toward us, hoping to get that big toe in our mouth because we learn so much when we taste and discover with our sensitive mouths! What determined, focused, adventurous, exploratory little minds and bodies we were in infancy!

We began to rock from side to side until the roll landed us all the way over on one side, and there we were, looking out onto the world on our side. A whole new perspective! As we tried to roll farther and farther, our faces, eyes and temples were gently massaged on that side. If we thrust our outer leg all the way over, we suddenly discovered we were on our stomachs, experiencing the bedding, blankets, grass, earth, or sand beneath our little bellies, and lifting our heads and heart forward and up in Cobra pose, we were lifting our little hearts up as if to say, "Look! I am here! And I am ready for what life has to offer!"

Rolling back onto our sides, if we grab the top knee with our hand, and begin to pull it apart and back to our center, we discover that momentum will carry us all the way to our backs again, and possibly to laying on the other side, where the sights are totally different. A whole new perspective again is right before our very eyes!

How wonderful and delicious are the new sights and feelings of the movements in our bodies. Oh, where our bodies will take us!

It isn't long before we are sitting up, looking around, observing everything with our senses. We are learning exponentially what it's like to be in this body, in these surroundings. Our legs, our pelvic floor, our spine, and our neck hold us up to see and experience all that is around us. The people who are taking care of us teach us about trust and nurture. We breathe in and we breathe out, using our bellies (our diaphragm) because it's the most natural way to breathe. Our breath is natural and involuntary, and it is necessary for life, pure gift.

If we reach our arms forward, and open our knees out wide, with toes touching, we find that we can lower our belly and our head all the way down to the floor. Resting in child's pose, our spine lengthens and we get a good stretch from the crown of the head all the way down to the base of the spine. If we lower our chest and lengthen the base of the spine back toward the heels, we get a good lower back stretch, and we feel supported by the ground beneath us. We roll our head from side-to-side, massaging our forehead and temples, getting a glimpse of the world to our right and to our left. As we center our forehead on the ground, that little pressure point in our forehead (our third eye) is massaged and activated, and we center down more deeply into our essence, a spirit being in this little human body.

What fun it is to lift the hips up and come onto our knees, and to discover that if we lift our heart and head too, and we lift up onto our hands, supported by our arms, knees, shoulders, and spine. There is a certain energy that is gathering in our core that is gaining momentum for forward movement!

It's decision time. Do we try lifting a knee or a hand first and then move forward? It's a balancing act, and we're learning what happens when we're on all threes instead of all fours. The motor skill coordination is being developed in our bodies and our brains. Lift a knee, the opposite hand, the other knee, the other hand, and soon we are off and crawling everywhere! We are suddenly mobile to explore and go where our eyes take us, so that we can touch, taste, and experience everything in our sight! No more just seeing from a distance, now we are on the move and experiencing more for our self!

If we straighten out one leg, and then the other, suddenly we are in Downward Facing Dog, holding ourselves up with our hands and our feet! We alternately bend the knees to stretch out the spine because it feels so good to lengthen. If we lower our chest toward the floor, elbows hugging in, and lift our hips higher, the spine stretch is even more invigorating. We breathe, and if we like, we can drop back down into Table Pose and start crawling again, or we drop down into Child's Pose, or if we're lucky, someone we trust will pick us up and hug and kiss us.

When we are feeling energetic again, we push from Child's Pose to Table to Downward Facing Dog, stretching out the spine and the entire body from hands to arms to spine and down through the legs to our feet, relishing in the entire experience of being in this body. And then we discover that if we begin to walk our feet toward our hands, we can actually get a different kind of release to the spine, allowing our head to hang down in a Forward Fold. We can even lift our hands from the floor and hold our elbows with each hand, releasing our head to let it hang heavy, really letting go.

If we then begin to rise up, we find we are standing in Mountain Pose, and the world looks totally different from "up here"! Turning our head from side to side we see from a whole new vantage point, and it's good.

Some babies don't experience the crawl; they go straight from sitting in Easy or Meditation Pose to standing in Mountain Pose. If that is you, you might try getting down on the floor, on a rug for comfort, and crawl. Go forward, backwards, to the right, to the left, and see what it feels like to be in your body, experiencing this specific type of movement. It's never too late! If it hurts your knees, don't do it—it simply wasn't meant for you. Always listen to your body. Your body knows what you need and what you don't need.

Standing there, tall in Mountain Pose, we might lift our arms overhead and stretch as high as we can, interlacing the fingers and turning our palms up to feel an ever deeper stretch along the side body. On the exhale we reach our arms over to the right, stretching the left side body. On our next in-breath, we come back to center, and as we exhale, we reach our arms over to the left, stretching the right side body. We discover how deeply we can breathe when we breathe into the side of our lungs and our side body. We come back up to standing and slowly float our arms down to our sides, standing tall in a resting pose, as tall as a mountain. It is from this stance that we discover the joy of seeing from way up here, and the experience of walking.

## The Human Experience

This is the human experience, the incarnate experience, and it is the same whether we are born into a Christian, Jewish, Hindu, Muslim, Jain, Buddhist, Sikh or any family. When I was learning this progression of our own human development in our bodies, my yoga instructor Don Stapleton, Founder of Nosara Yoga Institute, excitedly led us through these movements, illustrating with our bodies that we are all alike. He smiled, he giggled, he laughed, as if going back to these points in time opened up a world of delight for him, and he couldn't wait to share it with us. I am deeply grateful to Don for teaching me the miraculous and humble process of discovering my body's developmental process. For more information on Don's explanation of the inherent wisdom in our bodies, his book *Self-Awakening Yoga* is an excellent resource.

The science of human experience applies to every human being on the planet. We all share these movements and experiences in our bodies. God made us all marvelously and miraculously. When God created our world, our universe, our planet, the animals, and our humanity, there was perfection inherent in all of creation. God made us all marvelously and miraculously. "God saw all that he had made, and it was very good "(Genesis 1:31).

The human experience also includes feeling. Some of us are thinkers more than we are "feelers" and this means getting in touch with our feelings can be challenging. For me, it's always been simply easier to keep busy and not take the time to feel what I am feeling. So, for me personally, becoming fully human includes the gift—and the challenge—of getting in touch with my feelings.

Recently, I walked into the yoga studio for a "slow flow" class. It was a hot afternoon after a long, trying weekend that had left me feeling depleted and heavy. We began in a restorative heart opener pose on the bolster propped up with blocks, and as I melted down into the layers of support from the yoga props, tears began to come to the surface. Sweet, instrumental music was playing that pulled me down into myself. My heart needed to express feelings of weariness and sadness and to acknowledge that my spirit was hurting. In the calmness, with the group collectively dropping into our own bodies and hearts, it was safe for me to experience my sadness. I was giving myself the space to feel, to release, and to heal.

I wonder if, when Jesus healed Mary Magdalene of the seven demons (Luke 8:2), he helped her move the energy of feelings that were stuck in her body? Could these energies relate to the seven powers of the soul's journey to liberation as Mary's vision in the *Gospel of Mary* instructs: Darkness, Craving, Ignorance, Death, enslavement to the physical Body, the false peace of the Flesh, and the compulsion of Rage...and as Cynthia Bourgeault points out, could they be what were later labeled "the seven deadly sins?"[88] Could the demons have been tied to feelings such as fear, dependency, sadness, depression, anger, resentment, and control (the ego) that clearly can result in stuck emotions in the body? Could they have been associated with the seven *chakras,* with Jesus releasing the stuck energy so that Mary could be healed and raised to a higher consciousness to become fully human? It is clear that Jesus understood healing energy and its power, for when the hemorrhaging woman approached him and touched his garment he "knew that power had gone out from him" (Luke 8:46).

The human experience includes all of the emotions, the movements, the thoughts and ideas that we have. It incudes our relationships with others, and highlights joys such as when we drive for the first time, experience our first kiss, get married, have children, and even the simplest pleasures like that first morning cup of coffee. It includes adventures such as hiking, running, walking, and watching a good movie. It includes attending a high-energy sporting event or dancing with abandon at your favorite concert.

The human experience for me is heightened by spiritual relationships that focus on the presence of the divine. These relationships bring the deepest joy for me. I am not so good at small talk or casual conversation, and sometimes this frustrates me. I am beginning to see that my heart is set toward talk of spiritual things, and while that is deeply good, it has never made me the most popular or made me feel completely comfortable in social settings, or even that I belong. I feel most at home with people who want to talk about God, the sacred, the experience of mystery, spiritual experiences, dreams, psychology, meditation, Christ Consciousness, the spiritual path, God's will, and wisdom truths. I enjoy a sense of adventure and travel in seeking out the sacred among many traditions and cultures, and I highly resonate with other people who thrive on pilgrimage travel. I call this sacred adventure of life engaging in "soul talk." This is all part of the human experience for me. What makes *you* feel most alive in your wonderful precious body?

## Being in a Body: Incarnational Theology

The joys and sorrows of the human experience derive simply from being alive. Inherent in our aliveness is that we are all incarnated beings. Incarnation simply means embodying flesh or taking on flesh. Christianity speaks to the person of Jesus specifically as the Incarnate Word, the Word of God becoming flesh, both fully human and fully divine. The doctrine of the Incarnation of Jesus affirms that Jesus, the eternal Son of God, took flesh from his human mother, Mary, and that the historical Christ is both fully God and fully man in an abiding union. This doctrine was formally defined at the church Council of Chalcedon of 451 CE, largely molded by the diversity of traditions in the schools of Antioch and Alexandria.[89]

Christians believe that the Word, the Logos, is Jesus. Logos, in Greek λόγος, as mentioned earlier in Chapter 5, means word, reason, or logic. This term was used both in pagan and Jewish antiquity, and in Hellenistic Judaism, and the concept of the Logos also came to be associated with the figure of Wisdom (Wisdom of Solomon 9:1-2)[90]:

> "O God of my ancestors and Lord of mercy, who have made all things by your word (*logos*), and by your wisdom have formed humankind..."

Philosophically, Logos goes beyond the narrow definition of its usage in the Gospel of John. Logos refers to ideas, images, associations, and thoughts being brought into the field of consciousness through the use of logic, reason, and words. Philo, a Hellenistic Jewish philosopher living in Alexandria at the time of Jesus, used philosophical allegory to attempt to fuse and harmonize Greek and biblical concepts. For Philo, the Logos is critically important: it is the Divine pattern from which the material world is copied, the Divine power in the cosmos, the Divine purpose or agent in creation, and an intermediary between God and man.[91]

In the Prologue of the *Gospel of John*, the Logos is described as God from eternity, the Creative Word, who became incarnate in the man Jesus of Nazareth, grounded on earth and in a historical context. Matthew Fox, Episcopal priest and theologian, examines the gospel writer John's cosmological description of Christ in the Prologue, and points out that Jesus isn't named until well into the Prologue:

> "Jesus Christ (that name is not used until v. 17) is celebrated in a cosmological context...The Word itself is light entering into the world and empowering people to become children of God... John is clearly describing a new creation story, one which echoes the creation story of Genesis in

its opening words, 'In the beginning.' The Word is with God 'in the beginning' just as wisdom is. The Word, therefore, is not only words but also wisdom."[92]

This new creation story gives us a vision of what is possible. The life of Jesus reflects a man who was born and lived with the wisdom of God. The term Christ in Greek, Χριστός, or Christos, means the "Anointed One." It is also the Greek translation of the Hebrew "Messiah." It was used originally as a title, and very soon it came to be used by the followers of the Risen Jesus as a proper name for their Lord, Jesus the Christ, and thus his followers came to be known as Christians.[93]

## Christ the Highest Consciousness

This title for Jesus, "the Christ," denotes an inherent wisdom, a reality that underlies all of Jesus' life, his story, his presence, his *essence*. I often wonder what would have happened had Jesus not been crucified. Or what if the resurrection had never been seen? Would he just have been another itinerant rabbi, teaching and spreading the message of God's good news, fading away upon his death rather than a force that began a movement so powerful that it changed the world? Would the title Christ have stayed with him? I think perhaps it may have, had his followers continued on in the teachings of his *life*, his *way*, his *complete reflection of God* through his very being.

Awakening to the experience of sharing in God's Spirit is the process of growing into the fullness of life. The incarnation of Jesus into a human body is the same process of incarnation for all of us. We all begin in our mother's wombs, some taste from the mother's breasts, and we begin to look out on our world with eyes of wonder. We begin to sit, to crawl, to stand up, then walk. We use our bodies to express our spirits. When we are young, we are open and full of wonder, which is why Jesus taught that we must be like children, open to the Spirit's leading:

> "He called a child, whom he put among them, and said, 'Truly I tell you, unless you change and become like children, you will never enter the kingdom of heaven'" (Matthew 18:2-3).

This Scripture is an explicit opening to understanding the *path* of Jesus: Christ Consciousness. Yogananda offers an understanding of Christ Consciousness in terms of childlike qualities as he reflects on Jesus' teaching for his disciples to become like little children. His interpretation of Jesus' words calls forth divine, childlike qualities in us:

> If any devotee aspires to be favored in God's eyes, he should desire to be the least and humblest in the world's estimation, utterly forswearing egotism and selfishness. He should outwardly keep his consciousness ready to be of loving service to all, and inwardly endeavor, as long as he lives, to contact in meditation the Christ Consciousness inherent in the Holy Ghost Cosmic Vibration ('my name'). Anyone who by ecstatic communion absorbs in his Cosmic Vibration—saturated consciousness the divine childlike qualities— humility, purity, love, joy—receives me; that is, gradually attunes himself with and manifests my Christ Consciousness. And he who receives my Christ Consciousness pervading the finite cosmos ultimately receives the transcendent Cosmic Consciousness that sent the Christ Intelligence as Its pure reflection in vibratory creation.[94]

As we grow older, particularly spiritually more mature, we can awaken to the realization that we too can fully become sons and daughters of God, that we can embody the Consciousness of Christ. It's there, if we are able to resolve and heal our own life issues of survival, sexuality, and power and move into higher levels of awakening toward a higher consciousness. It's available to us after our lower chakra needs are met and we are able to spiritually "grow up" into the truth. As Cynthia Bourgeault so wisely says of Christianity, "An essential incarnational principle at the heart of Christianity is the unbreakable continuity between the divine archetype and its human embodiment."[95] This is the I AM in each of us.

## Word Made Flesh

When I taught my first yoga class in Nosara, Costa Rica, I asked my class to place their hands in prayer position and bow their heads, in prayer, to the divine. We entered into three-part breath, and then I offered, "In the beginning was the Word, and the Word was with God, and the Word was God." Our prayer had begun...on our mats, in our bodies, through our movement, our breath, our word.

We then chanted the word Aum, or Om, the cosmic sound vibration, and the first word spoken by a baby. Interestingly, in the Hindu religion, this cosmic sound vibration is the absolute *Brahman* offered as sound. *Brahman* for the Hindu is the name for the unmanifest supreme consciousness, God. This sound is supreme consciousness, a connection with the divine, which we bring to sound through our own bodies and voices. For Christians, sound doesn't seem to adequately fulfill the holy and mighty likeness of God as we know from our Scriptures, but can we creatively use our imagination to hear and possibly feel the vibratory primal sound of God speaking creation into existence? Can that sound be the movement of consciousness?

In his life, Jesus embodied a spirit of supreme consciousness. For Jesus' early followers, it was indeed the resurrection that changed everything. According to the *Gospel of Mary*, both in his life and his resurrection, Jesus opened up a mystical path of seeing and knowing the presence of God within that his followers could achieve.

For his early followers, as we know from the canonical Scriptures, it was the resurrection that changed everything. However difficult it may be to truly imagine the resurrection, this event was the catalyst for Jesus' followers to undergo an even greater commitment to continue telling the stories of his life and teachings and for their own deeper transformation to align with his path. And yet, the *Gospel of Mary* presents a set of teachings that make possible a path to a higher spiritual consciousness, and could it be that this path reflected his life, and then ultimately his resurrection? Cynthia Bourgeault, Episcopal priest, describes the impact of his presence:

> The earliest Christians experienced Jesus as *present*: alive, palpable, vibrantly connected; their experience was that the walls between the realms are paper thin and that our embodiment is no obstacle to the full and intimate participation in relationship with him here and now. The kingdom of heaven is not later, it is *lighter:* it exists right here, right beneath our noses, in a more subtle but expansive presence that is ours the moment we move beyond our egoically generated space-time continuum (what Jesus calls 'the world") and directly encounter the Source. From this imaginal plane of reality, reality floods back into our own world and fills us with grace, presence, and creativity. Here we discover that God is not only for us, but *with* us.

The earliest Christians awakened to this reality at the resurrection; this was in fact the *real* resurrection—not the resuscitation of a body that later tradition would come to set such store by, but the unmistakable certainty that Jesus was present and that their hearts now knew their way to him... And as the Gospel of Mary Magdalene makes clear, whether this encounter takes the form of a vision, an intuition, or a physical reunion, the real meeting ground is in the imaginal.[96]

For Bourgeault, imaginal does not mean "imaginary" such as fictitious or subjective. It means the realm in which images—the eternal prototypes—reveal themselves in their full authenticity.[97] If she is right, which I suspect she is, Bourgeault is affirming the possibility that we can have a direct encounter with God that gives us an awareness that the risen Christ is fully present to us when we are in our bodies and open to a mystical experience. To have a mystical experience of God, our human bodies participate when we open our hearts to receive the gift of communion of our spirit with Christ's Spirit and to recognize our own *imago Dei* that we share with him.

Thich Nhat Hanh describes the tradition from an Asian perspective that mirrors the idea that we are created in God's image, and then goes further to explain spirituality inclusive of the body:

> In the Greek Orthodox church, the idea of deification, that a person is a microcosm of God, is very inspiring. It is close to the Asian tradition that states that the body of a human being is a minicosmos. God made humans so that humans can become God. A human being is a mini-God, a *micro-theos* who has been created in order to

participate in the divinity of God. Deification is made not only of the spirit but of the body of a human also.[98]

In the *Gospel of Philip*, St. Philip also affirms the body as integral to spirituality: *"Sacred beings are entirely holy, including their bodies"*[99] (Analogue 60).

When I lead YogaMass and yoga classes, it is important to me to use Christian language and prayer to make the connection that we are made in the image of God and to invite Christ Consciousness into our experience. The Word of God is here, mystically, with us and within us, and being spoken through us: *Aum*. The Word of God is alive, present, still flowing, still creating—among us, within us, and through us. We are the Body of Christ, the living presence of God's creative energy, longing to return to our source, to God, from whom all things are made.

Our spirits long to come home, to the God who created our very being. Thomas Merton describes our center in God so beautifully in *Conjectures of a Guilty Bystander*:

> At the center of our being is a point of nothingness which is untouched by sin and by illusion, a point of pure truth, a point or spark which belongs entirely to God, which is never at our disposal...It is like a pure diamond, blazing with the invisible light of heaven. It is in everybody, and if we could see it we would see these billions of points of light coming together in the face and blaze of a sun that would make all the darkness and cruelty of life vanish completely...I have no program for this seeing. It is only given. But the gate of heaven is everywhere.[100]

I often wonder what it would be like if we could see the billions of points of light in each other as we breathe, smile, move, talk, touch, and feel. Picture in your mind the image of all the technological network nodes of communications and waves happening all over the world globally. Imagine our bodies filled with those same types of lights that we can connect and flow to each other in communication and love. The practice of yoga and meditation helps me to see this reality, and to imagine the possibility that someday we can all realize our connections as embodied points of light. The more people can visualize our bodies filled with these bright lights, the more we will manifest our light into reality—the incarnation of God's lights, God's Spirits with our spirits, made visible *through our bodies, minds, and souls.* This will be the kingdom of Heaven on earth.

## Embodied Spirituality

Our bodies, in addition to being the vessels for these points of light within our spirits, belong to God, and are made of God's creation, of the minerals and substances of the earth. In the Episcopal Church during our Ash Wednesday service at the start of the Lenten season each year, we set our intention to remember that we are made of God's creation, Mother Earth: *"Remember that you are dust, and to dust you shall return"* (Book of Common Prayer).

Cyprian Consiglio describes so beautifully our interconnectedness with the earth and all of creation:

> "As body, we are part of the earth, and just like all of reality, the physical organism of our body is a structure of energies through which *we are part of the physical universe,* connected to every element of creation from the beginning of time."[101]

We are reflections of God's image, and it would be shortsighted of us to imagine that this only applies to one aspect of ourselves, the spirit. Richard Rohr explains how our bodies have been minimized and treated negatively in the Christian faith:

> Apart from a general Platonic denial of the body in most religions, Paul made a most unfortunate choice of the word *flesh* as the very enemy of *Spirit* (for example, Galatians 5:16-24). Now we would probably say 'ego' or 'small self,' which would be much closer to his actual intended meaning. Remember that Christianity is the religion that believes 'the Word became flesh' (John 1:13), and Jesus even returned to the 'flesh' after the Resurrection (Luke 24:40)—so flesh cannot be bad for us. If Christianity is in any way anti-body, it is never authentic Christianity. Merton rightly recognized that it was not the body that had to 'die' but the 'false self' that we do not need anyway. It becomes a too-easy substitute for our deeper and deepest truth.[102]

Becoming fully alive in this body is key when on the path of awakening as a spiritually realized human being. It is through these bodies—our souls looking out through our eyes to feast on God's creation, and through all of our senses—that we have the privilege of bringing the divine reflection onto this earth, and we *get to* experience life as a human being. Within the body, our souls and spirits breathe and move and feel fully alive, and we reflect the divine image of God *through* us, *outward* into the world. By reflecting the divine image of Christ's consciousness into our daily, incarnated experience, we elevate our soul's existence and the entire community around us (and by contrast, when we don't, the community and/or world around us is impacted negatively relative to our sphere of influence).

Our soul consciousness grows in many ways through our prayers and intention, our study, our worship, our service, and our relationships, and it is in our incarnated bodies that we are blessed to have the opportunity to make a difference, and to grow our souls into the consciousness of Christ. Ultimately, the state of our souls is reflected in what we do in this life, how we treat others, how we relate to ourselves, to God, to others and to all of creation—and the state of our soul impacts how we carry on in our soul-state after we die. Christians refer to the afterlife as heaven or hell, and I am convinced that heaven or hell is right here, right now, based on our actions and our relationships. Eternal life is now, while we are alive, and it includes death too, but the spiritual life calls us to pay attention to the now, to be fully present to God in this very moment. Our spiritual task, as we raise our consciousness, is to participate in the raising of the consciousness of all others, for we are truly all in this life together, one global human race.

St. Paul teaches us to be intentional about our spirituality while in these bodies: "If we live by the Spirit, let us also walk by the Spirit" (Galatians 5:25). I am drawn to the notion of "walking in the spirit." For me, it implies more than just a metaphor of life in the Spirit, but also the real and palpable movement using our bodies, "walking." When we approach our spiritual life in an embodied way, we pay attention to the incarnation of our souls and the divine spark within into these particular bodies that allow us to enjoy life on this planet, experiencing movement and engagement with the world around us. When we pray the words of the Lord's Prayer, we pray for the heart of God: "Thy kingdom come, thy will be done, on earth as it is in heaven." My heart sees "*on earth*" as an inclusive term along with the plants, trees, animals, the ground and all that is made of the elements of the earth. "The earth" includes my body and your body.

On my mat, giving full, undivided attention to breath and movement—going to my edge and sometimes backing off intentionally—brings me again and again into the awareness of my spirit *within* my body. Not *instead* of my body, but *within* my body. With this body, created by God, I am an embodiment of God's light, and I can reflect the light of Christ Consciousness. I just needed to discover it, then believe it, and most importantly, live it. Even if we don't quite believe we can reflect Christ Consciousness, we can practice it, until one day when we realize "I am That Too," as Thich Nhat Hanh wrote about, if even for a moment.

Yes, I am that. I am earth. I am water. I am stardust. I am the dust of the holy One. God is in me, and I am in God. As it was in the beginning is now and ever shall be, world without end. Amen.

# ~9~

# Living in the Flow –
## *Surrender*

One must be able to let things happen.

*−Carl Jung*[103]

## Surrender is a Spiritual Practice

The practice of surrender is what allows us to make room for what God is doing in our lives. It is in the letting go that we give God space to create something new with our lives. The *Tao Te Ching* teaches: "Shape clay into a vessel; it is the space within that makes it useful." The practice of surrender is also what allows us to flow with God, aware of, and connected to, the divine spark of God within leading us forward.

Fully flowing in the Spirit of God means letting go of attachments, not necessarily physically letting go but as an inner state of surrender. Deborah Adele, yoga educator and author, describes how deadly it can be when we remain attached to objects and possessions. Holding on too closely isn't good for us, and she illustrates this by telling the story of the ancient way of capturing monkeys in India:

> In the process of catching monkeys, small cages with narrow bars are made and a banana is placed inside the cage. The monkeys come along, reach in between the bars, and grab the banana. Then

the monkeys begin the impossible task of trying to pull the banana through the bars. And here is the amazing thing—in the moment when the monkey catchers come along, the monkeys are totally free. There is nothing keeping them from running off to safety as they hear danger approach. All they have to do it to let go of the banana. Instead, they refuse to release the banana and are easily taken into captivity.[104]

This story evokes sadness in me for the innocent and unknowing monkeys. And I feel sad for we humans as well, because like the monkeys, we don't know what we don't know. How easy it would be for them to be free. The same is true for us; how easy it would be for us to be free of the burdens that weigh us down, if we could simply let go and not hold on. This applies to material possessions, money, and even people, when we are in relationships that aren't good for us. It's a call to let go, release from clinging, and share what we have, even give it away. It is in the letting go and the setting free of what we cling to that we too become free.

I know a woman who had many possessions, who lived in a very nice house in a very nice neighborhood, but she was too afraid to leave the house for fear that someone would break in and take her nice things. Her possessions owned her, instead of her owning them. That is not freedom and it does not bring peace.

Some of the happiest and most peaceful people I know have very little in the way of possessions. In northern Mexico, just across the US border, I met a couple that lived in a small house with an adjoining kitchen. A group of us from the seminary were on an educational trip for multi-cultural ministry, and we visited this couple. They shared what they had: homemade tortillas with *pica de gallo* and refried beans. It was simple, but it was a feast. They shared what they had with our large group out of generosity and abundance, not scarcity. They gave much from so little possessions. We left their home satisfied and renewed, in heart and in soul.

My yoga teacher Robert Boustany teaches, "Letting go implies that we have to *not* hold on. We must let go of everything, especially heartaches." Heartaches are dangerous, they will kill you, either physical or spiritually or both. We must let them go. When we don't let go, our bodies store the painful memories and emotions, creating imbalance and eventually dis-ease. Scripturally, Jesus taught the importance of letting go when Mary Magdalene, who loved him deeply, encountered him in the garden in the early morning after his resurrection (John 20:17). He told her, "Do not hold on to me." Letting go was essential—for his sake, for God's sake, for her sake. When we learn to embrace what we would rather deny, we surrender to "what is." That is the only path to living fully and freely.

We must release the stuck energy of our memories and emotions, using prayer and yoga and meditation, for our healing. A wise person once told me as I was flowing in yoga *asanas* on my mat, "Let go of what no longer serves you." When we release what doesn't serve us anymore, we allow space for God to do something altogether new. *That is why surrender is a spiritual practice.* When we let go, we open to God's next new thing or creation for us. As hard as it is to let go, there is a blessing unfolding that we simply can't yet see. We have to let go and trust. Letting go is necessary for us to flow with life in God.

Benedictine Sister Joan Chittister tells a Zen story of the freedom that comes from letting go:

> Two monks were walking down a muddy, rain-logged road on the way back to their monastery after a morning of begging. They saw a beautiful young girl standing beside a large deep puddle unable to get across without ruining her clothes. The first monk, seeing the situation, offered to carry the girl to the other side, though monks

had nothing whatsoever to do with women. The second monk was astonished at the act but said nothing about it for hours. Finally, at the end of the day, he said to his companion, 'I want to talk to you about that girl.' And the first monk said, 'Dear brother, are you still carrying that girl? I put her down hours ago.'[105]

## Being Free in the Moment

One way to surrender is to learn to be present in the moment, fully aware of the experience. This requires releasing the emotions associated with events or relationships of the past and the worries and desires of the future. When we focus on the past or the future, we miss the joy of being present in this moment. We miss the gift of life that is right here, right now, in this body and with this breath. Surrendering into the moment with awareness helps us to relax into "what is," which really is all there is when we are experiencing it, isn't it? We can choose to waste the present by dwelling on the past or anticipating the future. Or we can choose to surrender completely into the present moment, acknowledging what it has to teach us.

Isn't it true that we can only take action in the present moment? We cannot take action in the past or the future; we only act in this moment, and then it is gone, and we are onto the next moment. The present moment is where all of life takes place, and where our spiritual practice is embodied. As I imagine Jesus living his life, I imagine he was completely aware of every moment, living into it and doing what he needed to do at that moment—for the situation at hand. Not worrying about the future, until that last night in the Garden of Gethsemane when he prayed for deliverance, Jesus simply stayed present and focused on the people he was with and the task at hand: healing, teaching, walking, breathing, praying, eating, teaching, breaking bread and sharing wine with his friends. His every moment was an act of surrender into the present time, giving it his full attention and awareness, with a deep sense of abiding in God.

One of my favorite mottos has always been, "It is what it is." This is a statement of accepting actually what *is* in this very moment. Acceptance may seem impossible in some circumstances, and that is when we must simply breathe. We know that when we are calm, we can make better decisions and create better outcomes for ourselves and for others. Breathe. It is what it is. Inhale, exhale. Inhale, exhale. Long slow inhalations. Longer, slower exhalations. Breathing is a powerful form of meditation for centering us into the moment.

I love this meditation from Psalm 46:10: "Be still and know that I am God." Be still and know that I am. Be still and know. Be still. Be.

Surrender can also be offered with a body prayer: a practice of *yoga asanas*, breath work, and meditation can be offered to God as prayer. In yoga classes, we set our intentions. These are really prayers offered up for our lives, or for someone else, that we hold in our intention, to be changed, transformed and made new. This is precisely what we do in prayer.

Walking meditation also helps us to center into the present moment for surrender into "what is." Thich Nhat Hanh masterfully articulates how to be in the present moment in his short, sweet book, *How to Walk*.

> When you walk mindfully, just enjoy walking. The technique to practice is to walk and just to be exactly where you are, even if you are moving. Your true destination is the here and the now, because only in this moment and in this place is life possible. The address of all the great beings is 'here and now'. The address of peace and light is also 'here and now'. You know where to go.

Every in-breath, every out-breath, every step you make should bring you back to that address.[106]

Shunryu Suzuki, the Sōtō Zen monk and teacher said, "When my master and I were walking in the rain, he would say, 'Do not walk so fast, the rain is everywhere.'"[107] Good friends remind us to slow down and walk slower, when we are alone and when we are together, so that our time can touch the eternal.

## Walking Meditation with the Labyrinth

Another form of walking meditation to help with letting go is walking the labyrinth. An Episcopal priest, Lauren Artress, rediscovered the labyrinth in the early 1990s, resurrecting it from the darkness of closed doors of the 14th century. In her book, *Walking a Sacred Path: Rediscovering the Labyrinth as a Spiritual Practice*, she brings to light an ancient form of walking prayer that has become a global movement across religions that "supports flow, not force; cooperation, not competition."[108] I highly recommend this book for any seeker on the spiritual path. Artress brings the importance of breathing into the walking labyrinth meditation:

> "Using the gift of our breath is not only a way into clearing our minds, it is a way through the anxiety, self-consciousness, or uncertainty that we may feel while we are on the labyrinth."[109]

She also understands the connection of prayer with the body. She writes:

> "Insights in the labyrinth are not always received verbally. One can sense something on the kinetic level that defies words. One friend of mine

frequently experiences an opening of the Hara, a stream of energy moving through her body that begins in the abdomen, in the center of the labyrinth. This experience helps her feel more grounded, more alive in her body."[110]

I first discovered the labyrinth in the early 2000s, and it had a profound impact on my life. For all of who enjoy walking the labyrinth, the walking movement as prayer sometimes brings answers, and most often peace and serenity. Some people have visions. Some experience God in a powerful way. Others find the prayer and walking movement itself simply must be enough for this time. Walking the labyrinth is like meditating, you cannot go in with expectations, only a heart open to the experience, whatever it will be. The Bhagavad Gita teaches:

> "Without concern for results, perform the necessary action; surrendering all attachments, accomplish life's highest good."[111]

I had two very powerful experiences walking the labyrinth while I was training to become a spiritual director. These experiences taught me to more deeply trust in God's movement in my life and also in others' lives. The first was not my own experience, but the experience of a woman in our group. One of our group members used a cane to walk. He found it challenging to walk upright even with his cane, and often side-stepped to keep his balance. Our labyrinth facilitators had spread out a large canvas Chartres-style labyrinth across the parish hall floor. We walked in socks and others barefoot, ten or twenty of us at a time. The man with the cane felt uncomfortable walking it, so he said he would simply observe. But we encouraged him to walk, that his sharing it with us would enrich our experience because he was a vital part of our group. As he slowly moved along the path, he struggled to keep his balance, but he kept going, one foot in front of the other. We kept walking in silence, sometimes stopping to listen to God right where we were standing.

After our walk, one of the women in our group shared what she saw. As the man with the cane moved along, seemingly struggling greatly with trying not to disturb others, the woman looked up and saw he was not alone. She saw a woman walking alongside him, holding him up and protecting him. In her vision, she felt this woman was Mother Mary. I imagine that Mary was patient, steadfast, and full of compassion for him, wanting him to have his own experience, a spiritual experience in his own weak and crippled body. That image made me realize that his body was just as capable as mine to have a spiritual experience in a human body. A different experience, of course, but just as real as mine. Both his and my spirit longed to meet God in our hearts along this labyrinth path.

This reminds me of a friend's mother who had learned the meaning of the spiritual walk of life's important transitions. Her aging mother was struggling with early Alzheimer's and had moved into her home. My friend kept trying to keep her mother active—chair yoga exercises, a walk outside to the mailbox, anything to keep her mom moving. Her mother wasn't in pain, she just didn't have the energy to move. One day my friend said to her mother in exasperation (although with good intentions), "Mums, it's important for you to keep moving your body—what kind of life can you have if you don't move...? And very evenly the mother replied, "I have an emotional life, I have a mental life, I have a spiritual life..." What a beautiful reminder of the act of aging gracefully and continuing to walk the spiritual walk. When we can no longer physically walk, our spirits can keep moving forward, closer and closer to God.

I also had a profound experience on the labyrinth on a different occasion, once again with the same group of wonderful people. At the time, I was a Human Resources Director working for the University of Texas Medical Branch at Galveston. I had heard God's call, and I had chosen to begin my vocational journey with a heart focus, by becoming a spiritual director. Our spiritual direction group was in the piney woods at the Episcopal diocesan conference center, Camp Allen, in Navasota, Texas, on our annual summer retreat. That Saturday night, we walked the labyrinth in the chapel. It was the same large canvas Chartres-style labyrinth, laid out on the wood floor behind the altar, with candles placed around its perimeter. The candlelit room, with the moonlit pine forest outside the windows, created a quiet, peaceful, and sacred space for our evening walk.

I walked the labyrinth and sat beside it quietly, in silence. Deep silence. I saw a vision, and in it, I saw a man, and he was lying down. A woman was rubbing her hair over his feet, offering a gesture of love, a gesture of caring for him and giving what she could in her humanness, to his humanness. This vision had movement and color; I noticed it was dark, like dusk. I was "observing" what was happening in this motion-filled vision, and yet somehow I sensed that it was *my* hair, and I was the woman. It felt unsettling, and yet I felt loved and accepted to be witnessing this scene, and to be in the scene. It was a very private moment, and I went back to my room and quietly wrote it in my journal.

The experience had a profound inner impact; it made me feel like I belonged, in some way, for the first time. To my surprise, the encounter continued beyond the vision. The next morning, on Sunday, our priest for the weekend, The Reverend John Price, led our Eucharist service. I have to confess, since I didn't "grow up" in the church beyond my elementary years, I really didn't know the Scriptures well. I didn't know all of the stories from the Bible, and even though I may have heard them, I had not studied them. The Gospel reading that morning was Luke 7:36–8:3, the story of the woman who anointed Jesus' feet with expensive alabaster ointment. When Rev. John read this gospel story, I was stunned. The gospel writer gives details of the anointing:

> "She stood behind him at his feet, weeping, and
> began to bathe his feet with her tears and to dry
> them with her hair. Then she continued kissing
> his feet and anointing them with the ointment."

This was my vision from the night before! Tears welled up in my eyes. And then I heard the conclusion to the story, Jesus telling the dinner crowd:

> "Her sins, which were many, have been forgiven;
> hence, she has shown great love."

Everything came clearly into focus. A feeling of total forgiveness, acceptance, release, washed over me at that very moment. My whole life—all of my choices, mistakes, and consequences—was released, and I was made new again. I didn't need to feel afraid or unworthy. I was forgiven and accepted. My life was God's now; this vision cinched the deal, so-to-speak. At that moment, I knew there would no longer be another way to live than to show great love, for I had been cleansed, forgiven, made whole, restored to God and to the body of Christ, the church.

That was the truth all along, of course; I just didn't know it. I had never been separated from God. God was there all along, waiting for me to rediscover the incredible love and peace and joy that radiates from the love of Jesus Christ. After a long road of poor choices and self-destructive behavior, I was finally set free, and that is why I eventually let go of my other "plans" for my life and chose to step forward in faith into spiritual awakening, into ministry, into life lived in God and *for* God. There was no turning back. Everything that had happened before was part of my story, and God used it to show me that everything was okay, that I am okay. My life, my worth, my belonging: all God's. That was the morning I surrendered completely. My experience of walking the labyrinth set in motion this major inner shift.

In many ways, the spiritual benefits of walking the labyrinth are similar to those of meditation and yoga. We are living in a time when the dawn of a new era is rising, and diverse opportunities for spiritual growth are more accessible. It is an exciting time to be alive, even with the critics of such spiritual accessibility trying to hold on to the older ways and methods that are quite simply uninviting for many spiritual seekers. The pendulum has swung. Lauren Artress addresses the shift from the Age of Reason to the new era:

> Empirical science has been the major proponent of 'If you can't see it and can't measure it, it doesn't exist.' This reasoning is beginning to be recognized as part of an evolutionary step we needed to take. But it offers only a limited view, which we have mistaken for the whole picture. The tyranny of the Age of Reason is losing its grip. The human intellect, especially when pushed to its maximum, is limited when not used in harmony with other human faculties. We must look for new models, new definitions, new ways of doing things, even for new human faculties that lie dormant within us. But we don't know how to do this. Without systems in place to keep our societies functioning smoothly, chaotic, misdirected energy is coming to the surface. The labyrinth can serve as a channel for this chaotic energy. It can help us forge new pathways.[112]

For Artress—and I believe she is right—the labyrinth can serve as a way to help us experience the energy within us, and channel it for the greater good as we listen for God's guidance.

Yoga as movement therapy can have the same effects and benefits. Meditation for awakening to higher consciousness, as the yogis have known for over five thousand years, also has profound benefits to the mind and the awakening of consciousness. This is not a new discovery, but it is a new discovery in the last few decades for many of us in the West. And yes, once again, it is all about *going back to the beginning.*

## Surrender to Balance and Ease

Our bodies tell us everything. It is an act of wisdom to listen to our bodies. Deepak Chopra says that our "whole body is a holistic, dynamic process in support of being alive."[113] He also wholeheartedly believes we can reinvent our own body through awareness and managing our energy. I highly recommend his book, *Reinventing the Body, Resurrecting the Soul,* for practical guidelines on taking charge of your life.

When we are happy, our bodies feel balanced and whole. When we are motivated, our bodies feel a surge of energy that helps us to move forward in the direction of our desires. The tai chi masters teach that energy follows thought. The energy in our bodies will move in the direction of our thoughts, helping us to reach goals. This seems to me to be a perfect reason why we would want to create positive thoughts rather than negative ones, and help others have more positive thoughts, for the peace of all beings.

Painful or unusual experiences in the body tell us that something is out of balance. Feelings of anxiety, loss of breath, pain, or other abnormal sensations in the body are warning signs, saying, "Pay attention to me!" Often, if feelings of anxiety and loss of breath can be attributed to an event in our lives that is causing us emotional discomfort (rather than a medical condition or emergency), the underlying emotion may be fear. Fear frequently causes us to "freeze." A common example is when one experiences stage fright. This freezing happens because we are out of our comfort zone and in a situation that stretches us beyond our usual presence in the world. Recognizing and letting go of fear is essential for restoring balance and moving forward.

One Sunday recently at church, we were preparing for our Sunday morning worship service. The music team was adjusting to a last-minute change in the service. The team had not practiced the sudden changes in the music. In spite of her exquisitely beautiful, soulful, blues voice, our soloist, Mitzi Coleman, came to me and shared that she was feeling anxious. She was having trouble breathing easily.

A typical response in the church would be to pray for the feelings of anxiety to lift, for her to have the courage to sing soulfully without fear. We in the church say to each other, "I'll be praying for you," and "I'm with you in Spirit." Of course I said those things to her, including the encouraging words, "You'll do great." But somehow those words aren't always as comforting as they are intended to be, and they don't actually make it easier or better for the person experiencing the feelings.

Words are helpful, prayers are powerful, and yet, I also know there is more. I asked her to breathe. She is a singer, so breathing with her diaphragm is normal and known to her as a technique for vocal breath control. That will help, yes. But I went further, saying, "Excess energy is stuck around your heart and throat chakras. We need to get the energy to move down and out. We need you to feel rooted. Would you like me to show you how?"

I surprised myself when I began to use the language of yoga and chakras. I knew that if her energy was balanced by releasing unwanted energy and drawing in energy when needed, she would be able to approach the experience with greater calm and ease.

This wasn't a difficult teaching to provide, and it proved helpful. First we stood in mountain pose, grounding the feet down into the earth. Using breath work, I asked her to exhale all of her breath downward, through the root chakra and down the legs, releasing the unwanted energy out through the feet and into the earth. With an inhale, she could extract energy up through her feet from the earth, travelling up her legs and into the diaphragm, ribs and chest. This is the three-part breath in yoga, filling up first the abdomen, then the ribs, and finally the chest with breath, and the yogic practice of utilizing the connection with the earth to become more fully grounded and rooted. I wanted her to feel how the nervous energy was settling into her upper chakras and that if she could bring it down into her root chakra and out through her feet, she would feel increased stability and fully supported while she sang. I instructed her to "ground the feet down and let the song flow through you, using your exhale to release out the energy that doesn't serve you, and your inhale to receive what you need to flow through you. You are a vessel for God's purpose."

As I knew she would, she sang the soulful song, *Gathered for Power,* beautifully that morning. This is an example of how the simple rooting and breathing techniques can so powerfully transform one's sense of "being," so that the "doing" becomes much more relaxed. I continue to be in awe that yoga and meditation can ease the symptoms of this type of anxiety dis-ease that we so often experience when we are called to rise above our comfort zone.

Deepak Chopra explains in his book, *Reinventing the Body, Resurrecting the Soul,* that centering actually is based on awareness at the soul level. He gives several approaches to meditation and breath work that can help when peace and calm is desired:

> Close your eyes and feel the part of your body that feels stressed. Breathing easily and regularly, release the disturbed energy from that part of the body. Energy can be released through the crown chakra also, by closing your eyes and seeing a beam of white light extending up through your head and exiting through a tiny opening in your

crown, or the crown chakra as known in the yogic chakra system. You can visualize your thoughts as swirling smoke that the beam of light gathers up and transports away. During a long, slow exhalation, the white light can stream upward and take all of your stressed thoughts with it.[114]

Teaching sun salutation, goddess pose, bridge pose, and other root chakra poses addresses the first chakra paradox to push down, rise up. Grounding into the earth, with the body, keeps us focused, disciplined, and present in the moment. It gives us a presence of stability and belonging, and shakes off (by pushing down) any unwanted nervous energy we are holding in the upper part of the body. Practicing yoga helps in the practice of surrender.

## Surrender into God's Flow

Demands on our lives continue to increase, especially with the advancement of technological communication. Gone are the days when a response to a letter or voice mail might take days. Today, communication is instantaneous, which means that expectations are immediate too. I hear, and even say too often, "Did you get my email?" In our fast-paced society, we are expected to respond immediately to every email we get, assuming we are all multi-taskers in the grandest of ways. This approach to the "fast life" isn't good for us—it takes its toll as anxiety in our bodies, as we frantically try to keep up. God's flow isn't chaotic; it is peaceful, orderly—all in God's time, as we say. The spiritual life is calling us to let go of our frenetic pace and to live more consciously aware of each breath, each moment, every manifestation of God. When we take the time to give our full attention to what is in front of us rather than trying to overdo and multi-task, we can become aware of God's presence right in our midst.

We may feel we can't let go; that is for the "religious types" or only holy people. The spiritual practice of letting go isn't asking us to live a cloistered life like the monks in monasteries, as most of us cannot or would not aspire to leave our lives and our families and live in a secluded setting. Letting go is about letting go of all that binds you, so that your heart is free. Letting go of attachments can seem like a challenging and daunting task, nearly impossible. But it's not so much about letting go of material things; rather, it is a state of mind and a quality of reaction to the events in our life. Instead of saying, "I *AM* angry (afraid / anxious / depressed)," a healthier approach is to say, "I *have* anger (fear/ anxiety/ depression)." This shifts the energy so that we experience the emotion but we do not identify *as* the emotion. In this way, we are better able to become aware of the emotion, to experience it, to let it go, and move on.

One of the best descriptions of surrender I have found is from Cynthia Bourgeault. She explains it so well:

> "The word *surrender* itself means to 'hand oneself over' or 'entrust oneself.' It is not about outer capitulation but about inner opening. It is always voluntary, and rather than an act of weakness, it is always an act of strength."[115]

Inner opening...of the heart...is a posture of strength. This is the way to new life, to offer oneself in an act of heart opening, of vulnerability, of love. It is the way of Jesus, and thus he offered himself fully as a sacrifice to show that love always wins. He was willing to fully surrender and die for the sake of love; his resolve was not resignation but the strength of his message of love.

Surrendering is the way to peace within. The kingdom of God cannot manifest within us if we are not able to find peace and live out of heart-felt love for ourselves and for all. At a talk given by the Dalai Lama, he explained so poignantly why surrender is so critical:

At the end of the talk someone from the audience asked the Dalai Lama, 'Why didn't you fight back against the Chinese?' The Dalai Lama looked down, swung his feet just a bit, then looked back up at us and said with a gentle smile, 'Well, war is obsolete, you know.' Then, after a few moments, his face grave, he said, 'Of course the mind can rationalize fighting back...but the heart, the heart would never understand. Then you would be divided in yourself, the heart and the mind, and the war would be inside you.'

Letting go—especially of a protective stance to save your life and your possessions—is not an easy spiritual task. But as the Dalai Lama reminds us, the cost of *not* letting go is even higher.

When we become aware of the need to let go on a deeper level, again and again, we can return to prayer, to worship, to breath work, to meditation, and to *asana* yoga. The benefits of prayer, meditation and yoga address the fast, frantic pace in which we live and help us to let go of the little things (such as rush hour traffic), and some big things (such as someone deceiving us), and the daily irritations in our lives that keep us standing still and unable to progress on our spiritual path. *Asana* yoga brings us onto our mats, mindfully focusing on our breath, and helps us release the tension and anxieties we carry, sometimes held deep within the body tissues and organs. Yoga helps us surrender into our bodies in the present moment. Yoga helps us reconnect with who we are, and who we want to be.

If your life is chaotic and frantic much of the time, then prayer, meditation and yoga can be an antidote, a medicine, for achieving balance. Balance brings wholeness, but only after we surrender to letting go and surrender *into* God's Spirit—leading us forward to whatever new thing God is doing among us and within us.

## ～ 10 ～

# Sacred Ritual –
# *The Eucharist*

Some of the best resources for knowing ourselves
are the myths and symbols of our religions.
–*J. Pittman McGehee*[116]

## Social Ritual

Yoga classes are rituals that express a deep need for connection
and feelings of vitality. A workout routine is clearly a ritual for
many: five days a week (or two) at the gym or on the running trail
without fail is a ritual. Rituals can be characteristic of ceremonies,
club meetings, and business meetings (think Robert's Rules of
Order). Rituals also apply to individuals as we engage in a series
of actions or type of behavior regularly and consistently.

For yoga enthusiasts, coming to the mat for a typical class
structure of breath work, *asanas, Savasana* for relaxation, and
followed by meditation is a ritual that invokes feelings of well-
being and gratitude. A typical structure of a yoga class offers a good
workout followed appropriately with restful time for integration
in *Savasana* ("Corpse Pose"). We come with expectations of
releasing tension, of experiencing ourselves by getting in touch
with our bodies and our feelings, and letting go of the baggage
we brought in with us. The ritual on the mat brings peace,
harmony and flexibility, helping to release the negative emotions
and thoughts we carry with us. We leave feeling refreshed and
energized. Sometimes we leave remembering that we are spiritual.

The ritual of having that first cup of coffee or tea in the morning is perhaps the one of the most endearing rituals for we modern-day people. For some, the ritual of standing in a Starbucks line is the routine part of their day connecting them to a larger community with the same "practice." Other rituals include cooking our meals, the ritual of preparing for work each day on a fixed schedule, even the rituals of brushing our teeth and standing on a scale. Rituals help us keep our lives in order. They help us make sense of everything going on around us.

Humans need ritual. Ritual gives us a sense of place, a sense of belonging. Ritual sweeps us up into the moment and grounds us in the present. It offers both a vision larger than ourselves and an integration into the larger whole. People create and express meaning through ritual. Ritual is intrinsic to our everyday interactions, including handshakes and hugs, ceremonies, religious rites and chants, theatrical performances, and rites of passage. Even a fist-bump is a ritual, which denotes, "We're in this together."

Communication through ritual is participative; it requires that those present become involved and play a part in the unfolding narrative. Rituals are an integral part of our human communities, and they were one of the earliest forms of storytelling when language was developing and humans were learning to communicate with each other. Roy Rappaport, known for his anthropological study of ritual, concluded about ritual: "I take ritual to be *the* social act."[117]

Ritual includes storytelling of the belief systems of a culture or religious group. Ancient cultures used storytelling combined with gestures and expressions in religious rituals. These rituals are powerful: they bring understanding and meaning of our human existence through remembrance and enactment of stories that help us remember who we are. For some, we remember growing up and attending church on Sunday morning with family as an important ritual of belonging. The rituals we engage in can connect us directly into sacred time.

## Religious Ritual

Rituals in the church are an important part of our lives together. Our rituals are a response to the mystery of God, and we gather to respond to that mystery through worship. *Ritual* is defined by the Oxford Dictionary as "a religious or solemn ceremony consisting of a series of actions performed according to a prescribed order." We also have rituals for our fellowship time, our social time, and for how we serve others, but it is our sacred rituals that define who we are as a community and how we find our unity. In the Episcopal Church, our sacred rituals are called Rites and are handed down from generation to generation in our *Book of Common Prayer,* inherited through the traditions of the Church of England and as far back as the early church. The Episcopal Church's Prayer Book rituals include the Daily Office prayers, the Baptismal Rite, our Eucharistic prayers, the Marriage Rite, Thanksgiving for the Birth of a Child, The Reconciliation of a Penitent, prayers for the sick and dying, and the Burial Rite— all rituals for sacred life transitions.

The rituals and prayers we enact are ancient and yet always made new by our participation. One thing I love is that when we say our prayers, other Christian communities around the world in The Episcopal Church and the Anglican Communion are engaging in these same rituals and prayers alongside us, making us One Body, One Spirit in Christ—a mystical and living reality of God in community. Other churches also gather at the same time to worship in their preferred ritual, offering praise to God. Imagining these collective voices is inspiring and uplifting to my soul.

The rituals of the church always bring me back again and again to the presence of God. God is already here, and everywhere, but it is the ritual that brings *me* into God's presence. Sometimes during the rituals, I become keenly aware of the presence of the holy hovering over the altar. In those moments, I am transcended into a reality beyond my senses, into something much greater than myself. The sacred rituals give me the deepest grounding in the reality of my life in God, in ways that no other act that I can participate in can do beyond yoga and meditation.

## Sacred Ritual

My personal ritual of meditating for twenty minutes twice daily is a ritual of grounding and centering my life in God. Reading Scripture and holy texts as a way of life with a set rhythm or pattern is a ritual. It is helpful to establish a special place in your home or a special chair set apart for this ritual of devotion of reading and prayer. A flickering candle, a cross, prayer beads, icons, crystals, discovered treasures, or other items placed intentionally to create sacred space deepen the soul's ability to connect with the divine, and the routine act of coming to that place where your soul feels the connection is a way of honoring your desire for that connection.

Every religion needs ritual to express the divine Mystery of their beliefs not only in words, or silence, but also in action. The church continues the sacred rituals from the earliest Christian communities that formed out of Judaism. Jesus was a Jew and participated in the rituals of the Jewish religion, which then carried forward into the earliest Christian communities. The Jewish people celebrated Passover as a ritual for offering a sacrificed lamb to God in remembrance of God's saving embrace over them in Egypt. The ritual was more than emotional or spiritual, it was also physical—an "embodied" sacrifice that people could touch and see. Dr. Brant Pitre, theologian, professor, and author, explains the importance of the bodily sacrifice in the Passover celebration:

> "In a description from the Mishnah, the ancient Jewish Passover focuses on 'the body' of the Passover lamb: 'Rabbi Elizer son of Rabbi Zadok

says...And in the Holy Temple they used to bring before him *the body of the Passover offering*" (Mishnah, *Peshahim 10:3-4*).[118]

The physical offering of the Passover sacrifice was a sacred ritual for a people to remember who they were. In Jerusalem on the night before he died, as was required for the sacred Passover ritual, Jesus celebrated the Passover meal with his closest friends. On that night, he did something outrageous: he met *outside* of the Temple, and he offered *himself*, his *body*, as the Passover sacrifice:

> "While they were eating, Jesus took a loaf of bread, and after blessing it he broke it, gave it to the disciples, and said, 'Take, eat; this is my body.' Then he took a cup, and after giving thanks he gave it to them, saying, Drink from it, all of you; for this is my blood of the covenant, which is poured out for many for the forgiveness of sins'" (Matthew 26:26-28).

His act instituted the sacred meal of bread and wine as a ritual for his friends to continue in his name, saying: "Do this in remembrance of me" (Luke 22:19).

## The Eucharist: A Sacred Ritual

The Eucharistic ritual became for the early Christian communities one of the acts of primary importance in remembrance of Jesus, and for the church one of the major sacraments, "outward and visible signs of inward and spiritual grace," as we say in *The Book of Common Prayer*. This ritual in remembrance of Jesus is the Holy Communion meal, or Holy Eucharist meal, also known as Mass. The word Eucharistic comes from the Greek word εὐχαριστία or *eucharistia*, meaning thanksgiving. In the Episcopal Church, as in other "liturgical" churches (liturgy meaning the work of the people), celebrating Holy Communion or Holy Eucharist is our ritual of giving thanks to God, remembering Jesus' life, death, and resurrection, and inviting God's Holy Spirit to make these symbols of bread and wine the real presence of Jesus in our midst.

Jesus knew himself completely in body, mind, soul, and spirit. He was human as God intends every man and woman to be, perfect in every way. Jesus is the exemplary model of human nature in his very existence, the *Super Mani* as the ancient yogis knew him to be. Jesus is The Master. As we come to share in his mystery in the Eucharist, we come also to be transformed into his likeness. As we remember that we are created in the image of God, we too can become empowered by God's Spirit to be like Jesus in his Consciousness. Deepak Chopra illustrates that all humans have extraordinary potential:

> "*Your body is boundless. It is channeling energy, creativity, and intelligence of the entire universe.*
>
> *At this moment, the universe is listening through your ears, seeing through your eyes, experiencing through your brain.*
>
> *Your purpose for being here is to allow the universe to evolve.*"[119]

If we believe this to be true and possible, it changes the way we view sacred ritual that is intended to bring us into communion with God. Ritual then becomes a vehicle for us to experience God in our fullness and to be transformed by it so completely that we become co-creators with God in our lives, and more importantly, to become participants in evolutionary change toward higher consciousness. Celebration of Jesus, and *with* him in his fullness, offers us a collective way into the mystery of God's essence in him and in ourselves. Bede Griffiths describes this ritual as one that "reveals and communicates the interior reality"[120] of the divine life present among us, inviting our full participation.

The reenactment of this sacred ritual of bread and wine sweeps us up in the movement of the Spirit, participating in a sacred ritual that Jesus asked his friends and followers to continue after he was no longer with them. Jesus clearly wished his disciples would stay together in community, carrying on his mission and his teachings. Jesus told them and us, "You will do greater things than I" (John 14:12). If we really pay attention to those words, this means that his work is not yet completed, that we have a purpose, and it is to share with the world the same Spirit of his love and compassion. We are told to carry on his Christ Consciousness—his *Way* of being—in the world.

The Eucharistic meal is also more than a ritual; it is a sacred dance in Spirit. It is a dance of love between the lover and the beloved. *Perichoresis*, the Latin term meaning "to dance around," is used to describe in theological terms the dance of God with God's own manifestations: God the Father dancing with God the Son and God the Holy Spirit. Just as the dance of abundant and overflowing love takes place within God's own Trinity, the dance of love also takes place between God and us. The love of God overflows abundantly to all of God's creation, and we dance with God's Spirit, integrating God into ourselves in a dance of praise and thanksgiving—pure joy—when we feast at the Lord's Table. God's Holy Spirit, God's life-giving energy, flows around us and within us. Yogis touch this energy through *asana* and *pranayama* as life-giving energy awakens and rises; Christians touch this Spirit through awareness of God's presence among them, in baptism, and in the shared Eucharistic meal.

The sacred drama, the liturgy, encompasses the rituals, the words, the music, the singing, and the prayers. In YogaMass, we create and participate in an "embodied" liturgy, expressed through movement and breath. When we bring the movements of *asana* yoga and breath work into the liturgy, we bring our bodies into the act of worship also.

## We Offer Our Bodies *and* Our Souls

When we come to the Eucharist, we come with all of who we are. In a dance of love, healing, and integration, we bring our whole selves to worship, offering them to God. We bring our emotions, our state of mind—whatever has been going on in our lives. We bring our past, our present, our future plans and dreams, our joys, our sorrows, and even our fears. We bring our bodies. *This is my body, given for you.*

This is not a new concept; in fact, St. Paul instructed us that our bodies are a part of our worship:

> "I appeal to you therefore, brothers and sisters,
> by the mercies of God, to present your bodies
> as a living sacrifice, holy and acceptable to God,
> which is your spiritual worship" (Romans 12:1).

Before we pray the Eucharistic prayer, and after we have heard the sacred Scripture readings and offered our prayers to God, the liturgy or ritual includes an "Offering." This is a very important part in the "drama" of this sacred ritual. This is the point in which we too do as Jesus did on his last night. We offer ourselves to God, in whom "we live and move and have our being" (Acts 17:28). In this offering, we offer ourselves, as Jesus did, a living sacrifice to experience union with God.

Many people think the offering is about money ("the church just wants my money"), and that's a part of it—an important part— the part that allows us to keep the ministries of the community going strong to share God's love and compassion with others. But that's only a portion of what is happening in the liturgy at the offertory. Depending on the ethos of the worshipping community, usually a beautiful hymn is sung, or solo, anthem, heartfelt praise song, or contemplative song. During that time, we prepare our hearts and minds to receive from the Lord's Table. We offer our minds, our hearts, our souls, and our bodies—the whole of our being. We bring our thoughts, feelings of well-being and of pain—every part of us—to God. We offer these bodies that we may have abused over the years with too little sleep, too much work, or excessive alcohol and cigarettes and coca cola and even coffee. We offer our beautiful, young bodies and our older, tired, ill, or broken bodies.

I offer my whole self. I offer my body, even though it weighs more than it did when I was younger, this body that I usually cover with a one-piece swimsuit now rather than a bikini (how encouraged and surprised I was to discover in the south of France that women of all ages still wear bikinis even when their bodies are no longer youthful!) I offer this menopausal female body that gets overheated for no apparent reason at all. I offer these eyes that have astigmatism and are back in glasses even after three rounds of Lasik surgery. I offer this heart that is tired and dreams of slowing down, hoping to find myself one day sipping a hot cup of coffee overlooking blue water and a white sandy beach, where it is warm and tropical and the smell of salt air permeates the senses.

In YogaMass we offer our bodies that have folded and twisted and stretched and opened with movement and breath. Our bodies are present and engaged by the movement and breath in the act of participation and offering. Because our bodies are active and alive with conscious breath and movement, we are able to fully focus our minds on what we are doing, and on what is happening around us and within us. The beauty of YogaMass is that the yoga *asanas* and breath work actually bring us deeper into the present moment of the sacred drama. In the process, we integrate our experience so that our love and our logic, our touch and our talk, all take place in a holistic way in this one sacred drama, this dance of love. We dance, we give, we receive, we love. We become one with the lover—at least for this moment—and we experience the abounding joy of being the beloved at one with the greatest love of all. As the late, great poet William Butler Yeats so poignantly asked in his poem, "Among School Children": "How can we know the dancer from the dance?" We come to know the answer to this question through our own experience: our bodies are not separate from our souls and our spirits, and they are not separate from the holy. This awareness leads us into union within ourselves *and* opens us to communion with God; what else can we do then but receive and give back with gladness and singleness of heart?

The point is this: at the Eucharist, we offer all that we have, and all that we are, to God. We give thanks to our Creator who made us so beautifully and perfectly, even in our imperfections. Our perfectly imperfect selves! We offer our complete selves over to God, in an act of surrender, because God is God, the Creator of all, and we desire to be as close as we can be in full union with the divine presence of God within us and beyond us. We celebrate the mystical presence of Jesus with us, and as Bede Griffiths proclaims, we celebrate "the divine Mystery present everywhere, present in the earth and its produce, present wherever human beings meet and share together, present in every gesture of unselfish love."[121] In our generous act of celebration and offering, we celebrate the divine Mystery present among us and within us. We offer to give, and in return, we receive. Jesus offers us his hand and his heart, whispering in our ear, "May I have this dance?"

## You Are What You Eat

You've likely heard the saying, "You are what you eat." The first time I heard this it was in reference to healthy eating and weight loss, and I understood it at face value to mean that some foods are healthy for me, and others, like Cheetos, aren't so good for me. That didn't actually stop me from a late night Cheetos binge, but I was at least more aware that I needed to eat healthier food.

When I discovered Ayurveda, the traditional natural mind-body healing system of India and the sister science to yoga, I had an *aha* moment—the realization that you truly are what you eat. In Ayurveda, the "science of life through medicine and healing," what you ingest provides nourishment, growth, and structure to the entire body. Our bodies take in food and drink, and what we ingest does more than feed us; it changes our bodies. Transformation from following Ayurveda practices and yoga occurs from the inside out.

As a Westerner, I am fascinated with the way Ayurveda offers an understanding to the way in which food feeds the body and gives life. Ayurveda identifies seven vital tissues that provide nourishment, growth, and structure to the entire body. These tissue layers are called *dhatus* in Sanskrit, and they include tissues in liquid form. The seven *dhatus* in Ayurveda are:

1. Plasma *(Rasa)*
2. Blood *(Rakta)*
3. Muscle *(Mamsa)*
4. Fat *(Meda)*
5. Bone *(Asthi)*
6. Bone marrow and nerve *(Majja)*
7. Reproductive fluid *(Shukra)*

Simplistically stated, after food is fully digested, the body begins the process of building tissues. According to Ayurveda, tissues form sequentially, beginning with plasma, with each layer building upon the layers that come before it. Plasma is rich in digestive nutrients and actively transfers these nutrients to subsequent tissue layers. In this way, even the deepest and most complex tissues are nourished by the foods we eat. An imbalance within any tissue affects all subsequent layers of tissues. Intuitively, we know that balance is necessary not only in our emotional and spiritual lives but also for the health of the physical body, and the science of Ayurveda helps us to understand the physiology of the body and the importance of healthy nutrition for complete and holistic well-being.

On the level of vital energy, Ayurveda defines three vital essences that control ordinary mind-body functions and keep us healthy and free of disease. They are *Prana, Tejas,* and *Ojas.* If reoriented properly, these essences unfold higher evolutionary potentials. These forces promote positive health and are the keys to vitality, clarity, and endurance. *Prana* is life force, or the subtle energy of air for breathing. *Tejas* is inner radiance, or the subtle energy of fire for digesting impressions and thoughts. *Ojas* is vital energy, the subtle energy of water, and the essence of digested food. When these three subtle essences are balanced within the body, cellular health and longevity are maximized. For a thorough study of Ayurveda, I highly recommend Dr. Vasant Lad's book, *Ayurveda: The Science of Self-Healing,* and Dr. David Frawley's book, *Ayurveda and the Mind: the Healing of Consciousness.*

As a Westerner, these Sanskrit terms may seem foreign and difficult, but the potential for healing imbedded in the science of Ayurveda is significant enough that we should pay attention. The more I study the yogic science of Ayurveda, the more excited I become about experiencing its effects on my own health. I am drawn deeper and deeper into the practices of Ayurveda and yoga in all of its forms as spiritual practices of caring for the temple of my spirit.

If I continue to fill my diet with unhealthy foods, then what is happening to my tissues, my organs, and my blood? What is the relationship between the proper functioning of my body with my actions and my mind? When my understanding of Ayurveda took hold, the depth of the statement "you are what you eat" took on a new level of intensity of implication. If I eat healthy foods, my body is nourished with energy, chi, or life force, and the digestive fire and water in my body are optimized for healthy digestion and elimination, and for feeding my body the nutrients it needs for optimal health. If I make unhealthy eating choices, my body will be deprived, undernourished, and will need to work extra hard and use up vital energy to "eliminate" the impact of my choices. And this goes all the way to the cellular level within my body. My choices have great consequences on my overall health and well-being.

The point is that in this life, we are embodying our spirit in a fully integrated system of physical (waking state), subtle (dream state), and causal (deep sleep state) bodies as defined in Ayurveda, which all impact our emotional well-being and our mental state or consciousness. A modern perspective is that the human is considered to be a complete organism comprised of four natures: bio-psycho-social-spiritual. Each of the four natures is inter-related and inter-connected and cannot be separated. Our well-being incorporates all of the aspects of our being-ness. A holistic approach to healing then becomes necessary, and the path to wholeness becomes life-giving and sacred.

## Eucharistic Meaning of "You Are What You Eat"

There is a physical, emotional, social, and spiritual aspect to receiving Holy Communion. We take; we eat. We receive spiritual and physical nourishment in community. In the Eucharistic meal, the mystical Christ is present and union can occur. The presence of the holy mystery is available to us and lovingly given to us, as Bede Griffiths describes:

"The eternal Wisdom giving itself to be the food of men [and women], the unutterable mystery of the divine love offering itself in sacrifice to the world in a shared ritual meal."[122]

Some Christians believe in the true presence of Christ in the bread and the wine, and others believe that they are symbols for us to remember him and to share together at a common table, where everyone belongs, in his name. The Episcopal Church teaches that in the act of celebrating the Eucharist, we experience both the true presence of Christ and the symbolic remembrance of Jesus. In the breaking of the bread, he is there in mystical presence. In the pouring of the wine, Jesus is with us in his mystical presence. In the sacrament of Holy Communion we experience a sign and symbol of invisible grace, and in my personal experience, divine Spirit energy flows, life force in motion. Thomas Keating, Cistercian monk, says of the Eucharist:

"The Eucharist received in Holy Communion awakens us to the permanent presence of Christ within us at the deepest level. The Eucharist, like the Word of God in Scripture, has as its primary purpose to bring us to the awareness of God's abiding presence within us."[123]

In YogaMass, as I offer up the consecrated bread and wine I say these words from the *Book of Common Prayer*:

"The gifts of God for the people of God."

And then I add, "Take them, and become them."

I am grateful to The Reverend Cynthia Bourgeault for her interpretation of the Eucharist in this way. She articulates the mystical and physical communion that is real and *possible*. Becoming the Body and Blood of Christ when receiving Holy Communion is personal and intimate, and it is about realizing the potential and ultimate reality of union with Christ: integration and oneness. And all those who receive alongside us also become one with us in body and spirit.

This approach is also deeply consistent with the science of Ayurveda. The offering of Christ's divine mystery is for us to receive, to embrace, to eat and drink, to ingest. We take and eat this bread, and we take and drink this wine, and in the act of receiving in love and gratitude, we take in both the mystical Christ and the physical presence of Christ into our bodies, in every tissue layer. The critical transformation is that we become what we eat from the inside out. In the act of Communion, we allow the mystical Christ to transform the layers of tissues within our very bodies and souls into the body and mind of Christ. We do this out of our desire for the ultimate goal of the Christian life: union with God. We want to return home to God, to the womb, to the heart of God. These are words and actions of an embodied spirituality, taking the very mystery of God into our own bodies to feed and nourish us and to become, as we awaken the body, soul, and spirit, God Consciousness incarnate.

It is a blessing for me to say these words when I offer Holy Communion, "The gifts of God for the people of God," and in YogaMass, these words, "Take them and become them," as I lift up the consecrated bread and wine, the Body and Blood of Christ. The gifts of bread and wine are an invitation for the transformation of our souls *and* bodies, both individually and collectively. I speak these words with all my heart, and each time I do, I am swept up into the experience of the holy mystery touching my soul and reminding me of the beauty of the gift of Christ Jesus for humanity. The holy mystery always brings me to a sacred place within, grounded and centered in my body and yet seeing the larger realm of the eternal presence and essence of Christ Consciousness in our midst, within myself and everyone gathered.

And then the people respond in the YogaMass liturgy with these words:

> "When you give birth to that which is within yourself, what you bring forth will save you" (The *Gospel of Thomas*, Logion 70).

This response is a response of authenticity, creativity, courage, and self-knowledge. It is a response that recognizes the potential for us all to rise into Christ Consciousness, his Way of seeing and being in the world.

We take in the mystical Christ, and we are empowered to become our True Selves, sons and daughters of God. Receiving Christ, we *become* Christ, and we are reminded that we are holy. If we don't believe that we are holy, then we are reminded that we can *become* holy. Communion at the Lord's Table reconnects us with his love and our passion, and the deep love that resides within us all.

## Do We Need the Eucharist?

I was one of those young adults who really didn't see the need to go to church too often. I had a relationship with God and I felt that was enough. After all, I prayed the Lord's Prayer every night, and wouldn't that be enough to sustain my relationship with God? After working long hours all week, I needed to sleep in and rest on Sunday, especially after late-night movies and weekends with friends. Some Sundays I still want to sleep in and not set my alarm. This funny story rings true with me on occasion:

One day a man told his wife, "I just don't feel like going to church today." She answered, "Why, honey?" He responded, "Well, I don't really enjoy it. It's not fun. I really just want to be alone. And besides, the people don't like me."

His wife urged him on, saying, "Well, I know honey, but you *have* to go, you're the pastor!"

Yes, there are those days! For most people, thoughts of staying home or going to the park or the beach on your day off are tempting. Knowing you can check your favorite yoga studio nearby on your smart phone app and choose a class that fits your schedule, it's easy to talk yourself out of getting up and going to church. And if your church offers a Saturday or Sunday evening service, even better! The self-talk is powerful and compelling: "I need to rest. It's good for my soul."

You may wonder why the Eucharist is so important to me now. It is more than simply because I have made a commitment to God. It comes from my deep desire for divine spiritual connection, and mysteriously, it grounds me in God's presence. And yes, I do believe that Christ is present always and everywhere, not just in the Eucharist alone. In meditation, in yoga, in nature, I can connect with God. So why go to church to participate in a Eucharistic ritual? Why take time out of a busy schedule to re-enact the sacred meal that to many people doesn't seem necessary anymore, or at least on a frequent basis? These are questions more and more people are asking, and they are fair questions.

The Eucharist is the principle ritual act of thanksgiving to God in remembrance of Jesus. Jesus said on the night before he died, as he was having supper with his friends, that he wanted his friends to keep having meals together—breaking bread and sharing wine—in remembrance of him. He wanted his friends to stay together, to keep gathering, to keep sharing, to continue on in his memory, to continue loving, as he loved them. The Eucharist is that shared sacred meal that Jesus asked us to continue, and "shared" means we can't have it alone. We eat with a totally eclectic group of followers from every corner of town—from different cultures, with different areas of interest and passions— because we love him. We are his family and his friends. And sharing the sacred meal together is the central act we do together, experiencing his mystical Spirit present with us, across space and time, in love. In that moment, we become one with Christ, one with God, and one with each other. We belong. The union we seek is made real for us, and we are nourished to go back out into the world to do the work God has given us to do. It is the moment that strengthens me wholeheartedly, and each time it makes my heart feel grounded, free, and glad, like the feeling of coming home. And so I return again and again to receive from the table of Christ, and as a priest, to consecrate and offer Christ's mystical and real presence for others to experience. It is one of my greatest joys, to bless others.

In a talk given by Richard Rohr at the Center for Contemplation and Action, a participant asked him to "please elaborate on why we go to Eucharist when we know that God is already ever-present to us." His response was based on an understanding that ritual is important to us as humans: "Daily ritual gives form and formula to life." The sacraments, outward and visible signs of inward spiritual grace, are there to help us recognize what is true, and Rohr expressed that with spiritual growth, we come to "recognize the bread and wine is a sacrament of what is true everywhere."[124]

Both groups and individuals need rituals to name and celebrate what is ultimately true. Celebrating together through ritual connects us to each other and to the truth of what it means to be fully human. We at Grace Episcopal Church Houston seek this spiritual awakening and connection with God and each other. Finding a community to discover this truth and live with an awakened heart is so instrumental and important on our spiritual journey because the support, encouragement, study, and discernment brings us closer to God, and closer to the kingdom of heaven that we seek. Of this kingdom, Jesus said:

> "The kingdom of heaven is like treasure hidden
> in a field, which someone found and hid; then in

his joy he goes and sells all that he has and buys that field. Again, the kingdom of heaven is like a merchant in search of fine pearls; on finding one pearl of great value, he went and sold all that he had and bought it" (Matthew 13:44-46).

It's all about life in God, seeing the divine in each other, and recognizing the divine within ourselves. Yes, we can discover the divine on our yoga mats, and then we roll up our mats and leave, having potentially experienced a divine connection, and we go on our way, individually, getting into our cars or riding the subways, disconnected from each other once again. In YogaMass, we experience within our own bodies, minds, souls, and spirits the opening, the offering, and the receiving together in community. And we are collectively aware of the movement of God's Spirit and the transformation happening within us.

YogaMass offers a participative way to engage in sacred transformation. Receiving the sacraments from Christ's table is akin to receiving from a deep well of Spirit. The Eucharist is about the presence of Christ in you, not only out there, but also within you and within each other. In YogaMass we acknowledge that what we are actually doing is fully opening ourselves to approach the altar to *become* what we seek, to see with the eyes of Christ Consciousness, to become fully human and fully divine. And we celebrate our *becoming* together in community—a shared experience of divine grace.

The words of Christ are spoken: "This is my body, given for you." As we approach the gifts from the altar, we too offer ourselves, our souls and bodies, to the living Creator God, ready to become bearers of the Christ light, reflections of Christ Consciousness to the world as we are given the divine grace to do so.

# ～11～

# Awakening into Christ Consciousness – *The Life Teaching of Jesus*

The real worship of Christ is the divine communion of Christ-perception in the wall-less temple of expanded consciousness.
—*Paramahansa Yogananda*[125]

## An Invitation

Jesus said, "Follow me" (Matthew 4:19).

Where shall we follow you, Jesus? Into the villages where the people need to hear your message of love and compassion, into the homes of the sick and dying and those whose memories and reasoning have declined, up onto the mountaintop to pray alone and listen to God in the quiet? Shall we follow you to the mountainside and share what little we have with the crowds, discovering that even our meager offerings become abundant in your presence? Shall we follow you onto the mountaintop where you are changed into a translucent, white glow reflecting someone who is completely absorbed into the essence of God? Shall we follow you to the banquet halls and share dinners with those of worldly views who may hear your message but not truly understand it, trying to meet them where they are? Shall we follow you into the smoke-filled bars and share your love with the people there, because you love them as much as you love us? Shall we follow you into the homeless shelters, into the prisons, into the streets where people are cast aside and forgotten? Shall we follow you into yoga studios to experience grace within our bodies? Shall we follow you to the depths of love, no matter where it takes us and no matter the cost? Where shall we follow you, Jesus?

If only we had your pure heart, your unfailing love, your commitment to wisdom, peace, and justice. If only we had your gentle eyes, your healing touch, your way with words, your way with people. If only we had your complete trust in God. If only we knew that we abide in you and in God, and that God abides in us. Come, Lord Jesus, *ma-ra-na-tha* (my mantra, as I shared earlier, meaning "Come, Lord" in Aramaic, the language that Jesus spoke). Jesus, show us your *Way*.

Jesus prayed for us to know the truth: that we have the potential to abide in God, in complete union with God. This *is* his message, a message of hope for human potential, as Jesus prayed to God during his final discourse in the *Gospel of John*:

> "I ask not only on behalf of these, but also on behalf of those who will believe in me through their word, that they may all be one. As you, Father, are in me and I am in you, may they also be in us, so that the world may believe that you have sent me" (John 17:20-21).

The unifying power of the good news is the abiding love that Jesus lives in God, and how important it is that we hear that Jesus offers that *same* indwelling relationship to his followers: a dwelling in God so deep that our hearts only want to be closer, more connected, and more intimate. We are already inseparable—we have simply forgotten. Just as fish swim in water, moving freely within it, and even breathing in that water to receive oxygen, we similarly abide in God—breathing in God, moving in God, living in God—the God in whom "we live and move and have our being." Our relationship with God and in God and of God is the true essence of our embodied being as spirit, in union with the Holy Spirit of God. Awareness of this true essence and living into it fully and completely is the embodiment of Christ Consciousness.

## The Consciousness of Christ

It is essential that we strive to understand the breadth and depth of the meaning of Christ Consciousness as it is unfolding in our societal transition and evolution. There are many variations and nuances, and each may shed light on the emerging understandings.

To begin, it is important we first remember the meaning of the word "Christ" in the context of Jesus' time. In ancient Greek, *Christos* means "anointed." In Judaism, the religion that Jesus was born into and adhered to, *Christos* meant "the Messiah," the anointed one whom the people of Israel were waiting for to save them and bring liberation. They expected a king, a savior. After Jesus died and resurrected, the prayer of his followers became one of remembrance and hope: *"Christ has died, Christ is risen, Christ will come again"* (from the Episcopal *Book of Common Prayer, Eucharistic Prayer*).

Today, many are awakening to the possibility of the Consciousness of Christ as a possibility for all of humanity. Yogananda, the wise Indian sage of the 20th century, in his commentary on Jesus' teachings, intuited that Jesus' highly advanced apostle, John, relayed to us in the *Gospel of John* that "all souls who become united with Christ Consciousness by intuitive Self-Realization are rightly called sons of God."[126] As sons and daughters of God, we too can awaken to the eternal essence of Christ Consciousness within us.

Paul Smith, retired Baptist minister, in his work to bring a return to the heart of Christ Consciousness,[127] compiled a helpful collection of sayings that speak to the many shades of meaning of "Christ Consciousness":

Christian author John Piper says, "Christ Consciousness is God-consciousness."[128]

Hindu Sri Swami Krishnananda says that Christ Consciousness is not the personality of Jesus but rather the God realization of Jesus.[129]

Matthew Fox, quoting Meister Eckhart, says, "Thus, the true self or inner person is nothing less than the Cosmic Christ inside each of us."[130]

Christian mystic and author of the groundbreaking book *Putting on the Mind of Christ*, Jim Marion says, "In the level of Christ Consciousness, the Christian is identified with his or her true Christ self, which is seen as in a spiritual union with God the Creator. At this level one can truthfully say, "I live, now not I, but Christ lives in me," as St. Paul said. The person with Christ Consciousness sees all other human beings as the Christ and treats them accordingly."[131]

Yogananda provides insight into the deeper meaning of Jesus *the* Christ, and Christ Consciousness:

> Jesus spoke of this [incarnate] consciousness when he proclaimed: 'I and my Father are one' (John 10:30) and 'I am in the Father, and the Father is in me.' (John 14:11) Those who unite their consciousness to God know both the transcendent and the immanent nature of Spirit—the singularity of the ever-existing, ever-conscious, ever-new Bliss of the Uncreate Absolute, and the myriad manifestations of His Being as the infinitude of forms into which He variegates Himself in the panorama of creation.[132]

"In his little human body called Jesus was born the vast Christ Consciousness, the omniscient Intelligence of God omnipresent in every part and particle of creation."[133]

"This Consciousness is the "only begotten Son of God," so designated because it is the sole perfect reflection in creation of the Transcendental Absolute, Spirit or God the Father."[134]

Bede Griffiths offers a beautiful description of Jesus' consciousness and its manifestation being a "spirit of holiness":

But behind all of his (Jesus') human experience of body and soul, there was also the intuitive knowledge of the spirit. In the depths of his being, like every human being, he was present to himself, aware of himself, in relation to the eternal ground of his being…At the same time, he knew himself to be 'anointed' with the Holy Spirit, the spirit that is present in the whole creation and in all humanity, but in him was present as a 'spirit of holiness,' the presence of God in his own essential being (which is what holiness signifies) communicating himself in love.[135]

All of these descriptions offer a way of seeing as Jesus did, and being as he was, and what is most inspirational to me is that this awakening is occurring broadly among many today. As the Spirit is moving, God's people are experiencing anew the very Christ Consciousness we seek. Some of us discover this truth in the church, and others are discovering this equally on yoga mats and meditation cushions.

# The Way of Jesus: A Life of Christ Consciousness

Many Christians who practice the spiritual disciplines of yoga and meditation begin to awaken first to an understanding not so much of the personal and intimate *realization* of Christ Consciousness as much as a glimpse of the *experience* of Christ Consciousness. Once it is tasted, it awakens a desire to taste again. The emergence of this new form of experienced Christianity through meditation practices is beyond belief and social structure, which are left-brain constructs. Rather, it moves us toward experiencing God and having a mystical encounter, which are right-brain constructs. It is an upward movement along the chakras, toward upper chakra opening. Social structure belongs to the lower chakras, and mystical encounters belong to the upper chakras. One without the other brings imbalance, and leaves us hungry for the components of life that we are missing. Belief without experience (intellect over heart) is an imbalance that can create a spirit of domination and the need to be right rather than a spirit of cooperation, flexibility, and respect for others who see things differently. Experience without a framework of beliefs can create a lack of understanding of what is happening and how it fits into the holistic view of life from a wisdom perspective.

A balanced approach indeed includes integration of belief and social structure as well as intuition and inner knowing. With an integral approach toward spiritual realization of Christ Consciousness, we can renew our faith tradition by going back to the beginning, honoring the beauty of all of creation made in God's image, once again "hearing the sound of the Lord God walking in the garden at the time of the evening breeze...and the presence of the Lord God among the trees of the garden" (Genesis 3:8).

Jesus, our model of the perfect, integrated, whole human and spiritual being—the fully human and fully divine pattern of God's infinite love—gave of himself to be a conduit of God's love, an energetic, living channel of God's love from one human being to another. In Jesus, God's divinity reflected and shone so completely and brilliantly, illuminating from him to all who crossed his path. He was indeed the powerful presence of God. And upon his departure, he promised he would send his Holy Spirit for us to live continually in his light.

The mystical Christ Consciousness is still in our midst. We are invited to become one with his way of seeing, his way of being. We are invited to become one with Jesus and one with God. The path requires full attention and awareness. Worship, prayer, meditation, and yoga can help us stay focused on God to fulfill the desire of our hearts.

Laurence Freeman, Benedictine priest and my Christian meditation teacher, always reminds meditators that every day, we start again. Every day, we come with an open heart to remember. This is a mindfulness practice, beginning again, in the present moment, in the presence of God. During meditation, if my sacred mantra falls away and I realize I am chasing thoughts, I simply and gently go back to my sacred word, and I am present once again to God. In the process of seeking God, I discover a truth of my very essence—that my being has always been with God and in God and of God—exactly as the Psalmist says (Psalm 139:1-4,13):

> "O Lord, you have searched me and known me.
>
> You know when I sit down and when I rise up; you discern my thoughts from far away.
>
> You search out my path and my lying down, and are acquainted with all my ways.
>
> Even before a word is on my tongue, O Lord, you know it completely...
>
> For it was you who formed my inward parts; you knit me together in my mother's womb."

As we deepen our relationship with our Creator God, we discover who we are in our deepest being. Christian meditation is a path to awaken to our true essence in God and then to embody the very truth that is Christ Consciousness.

Yogic meditation also takes us to the awakening of our true essence. As taught by Patanjali, yogic meditation outlines various stages of meditation, which ultimately lead to *Samadhi*, or union with God. The first stage is meditation, concentration of the mind, or *Dharana* in Sanskrit. In this stage, we say our mantra and when we fall off, we keep coming back to it. The next stage, which may take many years to actualize, is *Dhyana* in Sanskrit, meaning absorption and expansion. The final stage is *Samadhi*, full integration and union with God.

The Christian meditation path fits comfortably in the progressive path of meditation as defined by Patanjali. Living in a state of *Samadhi* is a full expression of the prayer of Jesus:

"Abide in me as I abide in you" (John 15:4).

The yogis call the state of *Samadhi* divine bliss and imperishable wisdom. This state seems to me to be what Jesus is inviting us to experience and to become: the manifestation of the abiding presence of Christ Jesus within us, in union with His Spirit, his Cosmic Consciousness, an eternal quality or essence. Meditators often describe feelings of bliss and inner wisdom. Could the yogic states of *Dhyana* and of *Samadhi* be what Jesus was inviting us to participate in, this divine level of wisdom and knowing? This place where your eternal Self is unchanging as it rests in God?

Yogananda speaks of the Christ Consciousness of Jesus as a universal Truth offered for the whole world, beyond the Christian tradition:

"Truth is meant for the blessing and upliftment of
the entire human race. As the Christ Consciousness
is universal, so does Jesus Christ belong to all."[136]

Yogananda is suggesting that the Consciousness of Jesus Christ
is an inclusive consciousness—applicable universally to all people,
inclusive of all cultures and religious traditions. This expansive
view seems consistent with how Jesus lived his life, reaching out
to those in need, crossing borders, hitting the streets, so to speak.

An ever-expanding view of Jesus' Consciousness is to view his
"I am" statements as the very essence of *Christ Consciousness itself*, his
Universal Self. "I am the Way" is that *Christ Consciousness itself* is the
Way. I am the Good Shepherd is that *Christ Consciousness itself* is the
Good Shepherd who cares for all of God's creation, reconciling all
back into the family of God, and leading us alongside the paths of
still waters to God who anoints our heads with oil and sets a table
before us. "I am the Vine" is that *Christ Consciousness itself* is the Vine
from which all of our physical forms and life experiences manifest.

When he speaks of "me," is it possible that Jesus is referring to
his Universal Self, the Christ Consciousness that he came to teach
in his life? Could his invitations, "Come and see" (John 1:39)
and "Follow me" (Matthew 4:19), lead us to a path toward Christ
Consciousness? Could he be inviting his followers to manifest
his level of Consciousness that brings into your very life and
awareness that which Yogananda describes Jesus as having: "the
Christ Consciousness within him was the same universal guiding
Intelligence of the Infinite Cosmic Energy that lights the lamps
of atoms and all lives"?[137] What will it take for us to wake up and
believe what Jesus said to his followers, "You are the light of the
world" (Matthew 5:14)?

*The Way of Jesus is the incarnation of God Consciousness.*

Jesus, fully human and fully divine, is our teacher and complete
representation of all that life and Consciousness can be: Spirit
manifesting downward into a body, grounded on the earth and

simultaneously Spirit rising toward the highest Consciousness, in complete union with God, the Source of light and life.

In the science of the chakras, Anodea Judith provides a framework for the movement of energetic currents that is helpful in understanding the movement of Consciousness downward into matter and upward toward God's Spirit.[138] This movement is "soul movement," soul incarnation. Physical manifestation or incarnation occurs when the soul and its associated energy move toward the body in form, density, and individuality, in a way that creates limits and restrictions of the individual soul. This would be a simplistic view of the creation and birthing process, manifesting in a human body. Movement upward, as a person's spirit moves toward freedom and expanded consciousness, manifests as the soul experiencing liberation with the potential to be set free into God Consciousness.

*The Way of Jesus is movement of God's pure Spirit of love and Consciousness into a human body.*

The Spirit of God moved onto the physical plane in human form, in the form of an innocent baby who grew into a young boy and matured into a man whose message was meant not just for his friends, but for the whole world. His message: God with us, *Emmanuel,* God among you, God in your body, the kingdom of God within you, God in everyone. That is why it is so important to love your neighbor as yourself—for when you do, you are loving God.

Christ Consciousness is pure love, God's love, for all.

*The Way of Jesus is that of the ultimate lover and giver of life.*

My spiritual aliveness really blossomed for me when I began to realize that Jesus was a lover—my lover. Not in the physical sense, but in the deepest, most spiritual sense. I came to accept that Jesus loves my very soul, my very being. Being so fully loved, unconditionally, and even with all of my faults and actions that had taken me so far from God, Jesus still loved me deeply, and was spiritually trying to bring me home, back into the safe, intimate, and yet vast expanse of God's presence. His love changed me, and it changed my life. Jesus gave me new life.

Have you met people who when you look into their eyes, you see the vast, deep universe in them? Whose eyes seem to be able to see through you and beyond? Whose presence brings a sense of the holy? I imagine Jesus was like that in every moment, every encounter—his presence was the essence of universal love for all beings. Absorbing his universal love in prayer and meditation brings freedom. His path is a path for the soul to find God while even in this body and in our particular circumstances of life.

*The Way of Jesus is freedom from fear.*

Ultimate freedom has no fear, not even fear of death. For death is merely a part of the process of life, and without death, there would be no new life. And yet, we are often afraid—of life challenges, of what if's, and of dying. When I have the privilege of midwifing souls in the last phases of life, I remind them and their families that as Christians, we say we believe in eternal life. If we really believe this, we have nothing to fear—not birth, not life, not death, not even the new and different life that is to come. In the words of St. Paul:

> "For I am convinced that neither death, nor life, nor angels, nor rulers, nor things present, nor things to come, nor powers, nor height, nor depth, nor anything else in all creation, will be able to separate us from the love of God in Christ Jesus our Lord" (Romans 8:38-39).

Jesus shows us that truly we have nothing to fear. Upon his death, Jesus became a resurrected body, soul and spirit, showing that resurrection is a possibility for us all. Birth, life, death—everything passes away—and then, miraculously once again, God makes all things new again:

"I am about to do a new thing; now it springs forth, do you not perceive it?" (Isaiah 43:19).

Before we die, we must live. We must truly embrace being alive, living life to the fullest, working through our fears to allow what new thing God is doing among us and within us to come out and be revealed. To embrace life fully is the Way, to *feel* life, to move toward healing and wholeness and new life is the Way. To be willing to move outside our comfort zone toward growth and new life in the Spirit is the Way.

*The Way of Jesus is to fulfill our life purpose courageously and compassionately.*

One of the more challenging components of the Way of Jesus is the path of "taking up our crosses"—which is a metaphor for us based on an historic truth—meaning we are to courageously face the challenges of life and do the specific work we came here to do, even if it means we will suffer through the challenges it brings. Each of us uniquely has a purpose, and an embodied spirituality that when fully aware, fully awake, healed and whole, is able to engage and fulfill that purpose.

Christ Consciousness is nothing less than the realization of our purpose. With both the intuitive kingdom of God within and the Spirit of God to guide and support us, we actually can do the most important work we came here to do. "Taking up our crosses" means we simply cannot rest comfortably in God's unconditional love for us, but that we become willing to spread that same love far and wide, in our own special, unique way that is our calling and our purpose. It may mean we have to make changes to clear and purify our bodies, our minds, and our souls, letting go of what or whom holds us back from our true purpose or calling. To do this, we have to love ourselves as much as we love our neighbors, and we have to love ourselves as God loves us.

Without "taking up our crosses" our lives would fall short in meaning and fulfillment. It is the specific Way each of us is meant to live our life, with the greatest awareness of God's presence and the highest possible consciousness we can attain. So we ask ourselves, "What I am here to do?" When we awaken to the calling of the spiritual path to God, we do our work fulfilling that call, and our heart's desire ultimately becomes the attainment of the mind of Christ, the Christ Consciousness.

*The Way of Jesus is to become Christ Consciousness.*

"Let the same mind be in you that was in Christ Jesus" (Philippians 2:5).

This doesn't actually say, imitate Christ, or be *like* him, but to have the *same* mind as him. This is a shout out to us from the rooftops, a declaration that his mind, the Christ Consciousness, is available to us all. The work of the spiritual path is to tap into this consciousness of the perfect order of the universe and all of God's creation, and to live from that awareness. When we embrace the passion of Jesus' life and love and we take it on as our path, we begin to live into Christ Consciousness.

To live, to love, to give from a deep love is the path that all great religions point to. The Great Emergence just may be the realization that God is everywhere and in everyone, and that Christ Consciousness is our full actualization into a fully divine and fully human being, regardless of what religious tradition one belongs to or what religion one is born into. A Christianity that inspires people to be transformed into the divine consciousness of Christ will bring more healing and compassion to all, which is so needed in our world.

A Christianity that transforms its followers into Christ Consciousness has qualities of inner balance of the feminine and masculine, of the *anima* and *animus*—qualities of balance that must be attained for individual and collective spiritual healing and wholeness. This Christianity values the voices of all genders, cultures, ethnicities, and nationalities so that we may be made whole and complete as a people of God. A Christianity of Christ Consciousness leads to the willingness to do the work that is yours alone to do, out of complete acceptance and sheer conviction of God calling and the faithful response with "the *same* mind that was in Christ Jesus."

This is the Way. May we awaken to this consummate potentiality within each of us, embodying and radiating Christ Consciousness through our words and our actions, and through our integrated humanity of body, mind, soul, and spirit.

## Singleness of Heart

Life has its ups and downs, its challenges of winding paths, as the spiritual path has its distractions. That's why Jesus said, "It is easier for a camel to go through the eye of a needle than for someone who is rich to enter the kingdom of God" (Mark 10:25). Jesus was not against wealth; he was simply trying to teach us that seeking more wealth and worldly treasures gets in the way of the spiritual path of seeking and loving God "with all your heart, and with all your soul, and with all your strength, and with all your mind" (Luke 10:27). Yet, despite the challenges and suffering that goes along with it, an awakened heart can say, "It's all good...it's all God."

An awakened heart has a singleness of focus on God and the true essence of all of life. It leads to a way of living courageously and stepping into your own voice, your own life. It is a way of letting your light shine—not just for the world to see, but to also be heartened by your light. It is a way of getting mindful about your priorities and how you spend your life, and focusing on what is most important. Some things will need to be let go of and released. Some things will not be as important, and the truth is we can't do everything. We may feel the need to please everyone, and be superman, superwoman, supermom, super parent, super grandparent, but we can't be everything to everyone. The truth is we simply can't be all things to all people.

Singleness of heart is about prioritizing what the heart says is most important. I am reminded of the beautiful, soulful, uplifting song by Xavier Rudd, "Follow the Sun," as he sings these words: "So which way is the wind blowing? What does your heart say?" There is nothing that makes you feel more alive than following your heart into its bliss, which is also your soul purpose, even with the challenges that come with it. You may discover this bliss in devotion, meditation, worship, singing, serving and helping others, loving, dancing, nature, walking on the beach—any way that gets you into this space of inner connection to your soul. This is the path, and it's the path that Jesus walked. He followed the Wind, the Spirit, the *Ruach,* which led him into his own timeless heart and the heart of God. And he courageously, gracefully, lovingly walked that path, with singleness of heart toward God.

We pray for singleness of heart in our Eucharist Liturgy in the prayer after communion, from the Episcopal *Book of Common Prayer,* that we may love and serve as God desires us to do:

> Eternal God, heavenly Father, you have graciously accepted us as living members of your Son our Savior Jesus Christ, and you have fed us with spiritual food in the Sacrament of his Body and Blood. Send us now into the world in peace, and grant us strength and courage to love and serve you with gladness and singleness of heart; through Christ our Lord. Amen.

The Christian path of discipleship is to become fully transformed human beings with open hearts: fully human, fully divine, open to God's Spirit or *Ruach* flowing in and through us, bringing light into the world. Through Jesus we see what a true Son or Daughter of God looks like, and what it means to live walking in the Spirit. My body, your body, our bodies, moving collectively as embodied minds and souls toward the wholeness Jesus shows is possible. Healed and loved, we follow our hearts into full participation of life in God. Fully integrated and awakened to our incarnate nature in God's image, we engage God's divine Spirit in the realization of Christ Consciousness, the mind of Christ—in these miraculous bodies that shine the light of our spirit in communion with God's Spirit to illumine the world.

## Seeing with Higher Consciousness

Transformation into higher consciousness isn't merely a goal; it is an experience that ultimately leads us to a Way of Being. We may or may not be preparing for it, but when it happens we will know. It may be a subtle and gradual opening of the eyes of the heart, or it may come from a sudden life event that sends us whirling down into darkness that teaches us a deeper truth and brings light into the darkness.

When our awakening happens, and we begin to move into a higher level of awareness or consciousness, we begin to shed the old way of thinking that we are separate from all else. This new way of seeing brings the awareness that we are all connected beyond the physical, and strips away the desire to win at all costs, the need to fight for survival. Jesus modeled that there should be no separation between our neighbors and ourselves in the ways we care for one another. Science also has something to say about our connectedness with our neighbors; in fact, quantum theory and Nobel Prize-winning Austrian physicist Erwin Schrodinger famously said, "Quantum physics thus reveals a basic oneness of the universe."[139] We are now even discovering our connectedness with trees and plants!

The transformation to a new state of connected consciousness is a beautiful awakening to a more peaceful and compassionate way of living. Rumi, the thirteenth century Persian poet and

Sufi mystic, a true master of the heart, so eloquently describes the process of awakening:

## This Is How a Human Being Can Change

There's a worm addicted to eating
grape leaves.
Suddenly, he wakes up,
call it grace, whatever, something
wakes him, and he's no longer
a worm.

He's the entire vineyard,
and the orchard too,
the fruit, the trunks,
a growing wisdom and joy
that doesn't need
to devour.[140]

Mystics have always seen through the eyes of connectedness, and awakening to this truth pulls you deeper and deeper into your eternal Self and the presence of God. Bede Griffiths describes this state of soul realization:

> At this point of the spirit the soul becomes self-luminous, or rather it discovers that it is itself but the reflection of a light which shines forever beyond the darkness, a light which is ever the same, pure, transparent, penetrating the whole creation, enlightening every human being, yet remaining ever in itself, tranquil and unchanged, receiving everything into itself and converting all into the substance of its own infinite being.

It is the discovery of this infinite, eternal, unchanging being, beyond the flux of time and change, beyond birth and death, beyond thought and feeling, yet answering to the deepest need of every human being, which is the goal of all religion and all of humanity.[141]

This realization, this expanded view changes everything. All things become new again, and we develop a greater tolerance for the people and the world about us. We discover we can joyfully sing the words of the beautiful hymn, "It is well with my soul."

This greater awareness of God's presence *everywhere*, within and around us, in ourselves and in others, is like a *coming home* to the simple truth of it all. In the meditation groups that I lead, using the teachings of the World Community for Christian Meditation, we describe the process of meditation, or the pure prayer of the heart, as a *coming home* to the heart of God. This is the path to higher consciousness through meditation.

In meditation, we release thoughts, forms, and images from our mind and allow our mind to rest in God's presence. As the mind calms down, we may open to accessing the sixth chakra, the *Ajna* chakra of perception and intuition. God speaks to us in this opening, and we gain a deeper sense of truth, wisdom, and "inner knowing." Our perceptions change, and we see the more inclusive aspect of nature, of God's creation, and we realize that we are but one part of the vast whole.

Suddenly becoming a widow after the death of my first husband at age 29 was a major catalyst for my soul movement into higher consciousness. I began to see that everything and every emotion and action belongs—as deeply painful as they may be—and that I was one part of this incredible and expansive networked web of life, energy, activity, movement, rest—simply, of this great whole. I experienced the deepest pain imaginable, my worst nightmare, and I also watched myself having that tumultuous experience. I connected very deeply with others in the same pain circle, and I could see that our pain was not exactly everyone's pain, but that we all have pain. The ebb and flow of life, of movement and stillness was so evident: surreal and yet very real; dreamlike and yet total awareness.

The spiritual journey continues as we learn and expand outward in growth and then contract and go inward, as we serve others and then take time for ourselves, as we experience pain and then heal. The cycle of birth, life, death and rebirth happens over and over as we experience what life brings—I like to call these mini-resurrections. They are soul movements of descent and ascent, cycles of the human experience that call us to grow spiritually in this life, awakening to higher levels of consciousness along the way.

As we grow in spiritual maturity, we acquire more knowledge, and hopefully we gain wisdom. We heal deeper and deeper layers of emotional and psychological pain. We understand the interconnectedness of our bodies with our emotions and our mind (how our inner talk impacts us!), and we begin to treat our bodies with the respect they deserve. We take on a more holistic approach to wholeness and healing, approaching ourselves as a whole system, clearing out what needs to be cleared, healing the memories, the experiences, the behaviors and attitudes that keep us in darkness. As we clear and heal, we become *lighter.* We eventually *become light* if we stay on the path to higher consciousness.

A miraculous integration of all dualities within oneself occurs as one transcends one's own thoughts and feelings to the highest consciousness: the Christ Consciousness. In yogic terms, this integration happens at the level of the highest chakra (the crown chakra), the *Sahasrara* chakra of the thousand-fold petals of awareness. Ken Wilber describes this integration and non-dual state:

> At the seventh *chakra,* the masculine and feminine serpents [energy channels] both disappear into

their ground or source. Masculine and feminine meet and unite at the crown—they literally become one...The two voices in each person become integrated, so that there is a paradoxical union of autonomy and relationship, rights and responsibilities, agency and communion, wisdom and compassion, justice and mercy, masculine and feminine.[142]

As the internal dualities dissolve, so do the external dualities. The experiences of expansion (*Dhyana*) and integration *(Samadhi)* take hold in our consciousness and our awareness. We begin to see with the eyes of Christ that we all are in this together. Energy moving—expanding and contracting. Souls dancing—moving away and moving toward each other. Bodies changing—new forms are birthing, forms are moving toward health or dis-ease, and old forms are passing away. All are interconnected; all belong in this cycle of birth, life, death, and rebirth.

Seeing with the spiritual eye recognizes that there is much beyond what we can see with the naked eye. The unseen forces are at work and play. In Christian language, the unseen forces are an expression of the Spirit, and yes, they can be an expression, too, of negative energy or evil. As Jesus teaches, we must stay awake. But we have a choice about what we focus on: we can choose to focus on goodness, gratitude, and how to make life better for ourselves and others, or we can choose to focus on the negative, living in fear and anxiety. The forces are present; we can choose to walk in the light of God's Spirit, grounded in prayer, meditation, and yoga to meet the day with gratitude and aliveness. The good news is that God is still moving and speaking among us. With the Spirit of God within us, and with the chakras balanced, consciousness rises toward the higher chakras. We begin to speak our truth more and more, we prophesy, we dream, we see visions of God's kingdom manifesting on earth. Just as in the beginning of creation, when the Spirit of God swept over the face of the waters, today the Wisdom of God continues to pour out among us as God promised, bringing many toward the higher Christ Consciousness:

> "I will pour out my spirit on all flesh; your sons
> and your daughters shall prophesy, your old men
> shall dream dreams, and your young men shall see
> visions" (Joel 2:28).

This spiritual rising happened at Pentecost, the birth of the church, and it happened again over the millennia and centuries as humankind has grown and evolved.

During the middle ages, Hildegard of Bingen, German Benedictine Abbess and composer of music and art, dreamed dreams and saw visions. In one of her twelfth century mandala art pieces, "Choirs of Angels," Saint Hildegard depicted nine concentric circles representing all of God's creation. In the fourth circle, the faces were so bright that Hildegard could not look at them, a representation of the body and soul of humans revealing the mystery of God and the incarnation of God's Son.

This work celebrates the human body and soul, and calls it into God's complete love, with a response of pure and complete service to God. This is an expression of God's Spirit giving Saint Hildegard a vision of God's kingdom, where all are called to move into the bright light of God. The sympathetic string of the "Choirs of Angels" mandala with the yogic philosophy is a representation of the opening of the sixth chakra, *Ajna,* the chakra of light and luminescent, of intuition, imagination, psychic perception, and clear awareness toward the highest consciousness.

This brings to mind also the prophetic voices of Patanjali, Carl Jung, Mahatma Gandhi, Martin Luther King, Jr., Mary Magdalene, and so many others, including the many teachers of contemplative practices and the spirituality of higher consciousness.

A new dawn is rising—it seems as though the awakening to another Pentecost-like experience is happening once again. We as a global race are moving toward higher consciousness, toward Christ Consciousness, the universal consciousness—even as an equal and opposite force is manifesting with great power to hold us down. This movement toward universal consciousness is a force that requires balance among all of our individual and collective chakras—the lower chakra needs of security, sexuality, and power demanding to be met, and the higher chakra needs of love, expression, intuition and union with God desiring to be fulfilled. These energies are crying for balance and healing.

We simply must move beyond what is best for the individual—or the tribe, or nation—to what is best for all. Christ Consciousness calls us to nothing less. Integrating Eastern philosophy, yogic philosophy, is an integral approach to this critical movement so needed in our time. Bede Griffiths explains why the bridge between Eastern and Western thought is so important:

> The encounter with Eastern thought, with its intuitive basis, is crucial. Christianity cannot grow as a religion today, unless it abandons its Western culture with its rational masculine bias and learns again the feminine intuitive understanding of the East....Reason has to be 'married' to intuition; it has to learn to surrender itself to the deeper intuitions of the Spirit. These intuitions come, as we have seen, from the presence of the Spirit in the depths of the soul. They are an expression of a growing self-awareness, of an integral knowledge not of the mind or reason alone, but of the whole man, body, soul and spirit. Faith itself is a function not of the rational but of the intuitive mind.[143]

As we strive for balance, which we must do on every level (physically, psychologically, emotionally, energetically, spiritually), we must balance the masculine and the feminine and honor the complete integration, self-awareness, and wholeness that Jesus achieved and lived. We must open to complete healing and clearing of our energy channels and centers, the *nadis* and the chakras, so that intuition and consciousness can evolve. Thich Nhat Hanh beautifully articulates how we, even people of every religious tradition, can move toward this higher state of being and seeing:

> "Every moment is an opportunity to breathe life into the Buddha, the *Dharma* [the Sanskrit word for teaching], and the *Sangha* [the Sanskrit word for community.] Every moment is an opportunity to manifest the Father, the Son, and the Holy Spirit."[144]

Every moment is a choice. We can choose a way of being and seeing that embodies an inclusive, embracing attitude of the heart. In his talk "Christ, Cosmology, & Consciousness: A Reframing of How We See," Richard Rohr speaks to the seeing with the eyes of Christ. Rohr quotes Teilhard de Chardin, the late French philosopher and Jesuit priest, who writes: "Everything that rises must converge."[145] Rohr explains,

> "Higher levels of evolution are always a movement toward greater unity. Along the way there will be differentiation and complexity, but paradoxically, that increased complexity moves life to a greater level of unity, until in the end there is only God who is 'all in all' (see 1 Corinthians 15:28). If it isn't moving toward unity, it is not a higher level of consciousness."[146]

A global awakening to the presence of the divine in all creation, and our inter-relatedness as a result of God's indwelling presence, is underway. Talk of non-duality—not this or that; not one, or two, but unity and integration—speaks to the increasing awareness of the potential for unity, an "all in all" consciousness. More and more Christians are turning to follow the Cosmic Christ who is the Word made flesh, the *Aum* of the original cosmic vibration, and whose Word is inherent in each of us. One heart at a time, the evolution of humanity into Cosmic Christ Consciousness is already underway.

The eye of seeing the interconnectedness of all things is the eye of seeing with Christ Consciousness. It allows mystery, it receives and doesn't control, it allows flow and doesn't resist, and it allows each to be in its own right. When I see with these eyes, I allow what is to be, and I welcome with gratitude all that is.

This path of higher consciousness is not a straight line nor is it filled only with comfort and ease. It is like a mountain road with turns and switchbacks, and the ascent is made slowly and carefully. Keeping your eye on the road ahead, there will be twists and turns and yet the higher the elevation, the wider the perspective. Each new view and perspective is part of the climb. The ascent doesn't mean we won't encounter suffering; in fact, the more we see, the more we are called to acknowledge and participate in relieving the suffering in our world. The spiritual path gives us new outlooks along the way. Each part of the climb is connected to the one before it and the one after it, and all are necessary. Nothing is wasted. Nothing is trivial. All is relevant. All is part of the process of being and becoming.

## A Global Higher Consciousness

The awakening of this higher consciousness in humanity across religions may have begun in exactly the process Phyllis

Tickle articulates in her research, the spanning of about one hundred years of change leading up to the major event and about fifty years after, until a new status quo settles in. Looking back nearly one hundred years before September 11, 2001, at the first World's Parliament of Religions in Chicago in 1893, interfaith leaders presented new perspectives that have forever since influenced our worldview in the West.

Anagarika Dharmapāla, Sri Lankan Buddhist, understood that during the nineteenth century, European scholars had reopened the long-hidden archives of Buddhist thought. As a result, he said, the world now faced "the dawn of a new era." Dharmapāla also noted how the rise of evolutionary science and idealistic philosophies had prepared the way for the modern resurgence of Buddhism:

> "The tendency of enlightened thought of the day
> all over the world is not towards theology, but
> philosophy and psychology."[147]

Swami Vivekananda, Indian Hindu monk and a favorite of the press and crowds, told the Parliament of a theological vision that was inclusive of natural and spiritual laws that encompassed God and the universe, as told by Richard Hughes Seager:

> The Vedas, [Swami Vivekananda] told the
> Parliament, were divine revelations which, unlike
> the Bible, were not confined to a single book but
> formed a beginningless and endless 'accumulated
> treasury of spiritual laws.' Like natural laws
> revealed by modern science, these spiritual laws
> had existed from eternity, but at various times
> they had been discovered by seers or *rishis*, some
> of the best of whom, had been women....

'At the head of all these laws, in and through every particle of matter and force, stands one through whose command the wind blows, the fire burns, the clouds rain, and death stalks upon the earth.' For Hindus, he explained, God was the everywhere pure and formless one who may be called father, mother, and friend, but whose greatest incarnation was the dark lord Krishna, whose grace and mercy revealed itself to the pure of heart to release them from the bondage of *karma*.[148]

"*Grace and mercy revealed to the pure of heart*"—is there a sympathetic string with Jesus' teaching? In the Gospel of Matthew, Jesus says:

"Blessed are the pure in heart, for they shall see God" (Matthew 5:8).

For the Hindus, the goal is Krishna Consciousness. Could Jesus be pointing his followers to a similar realization, but of Christ Consciousness? Could the different teachings between these religions be pointing to the universal truth of supreme Cosmic Consciousness? Could this be the meaning of Jesus' teaching: "The kingdom of God is among you" (Luke 17:21)? Some translations of the Holy Bible (including the New Revised Standard Version in footnote) use the word "within" instead of "among." The word choice changes everything for me. Could the kingdom of God be the awareness of the highest Christ Consciousness available to you and me?

At the Parliament, Swami Vivekananda explained that the goal of Hinduism is union with God Consciousness:

[Hinduism] did not consist of dogmas, doctrines, or creeds, but 'in being and becoming;' its goal was to unite the soul with the universal consciousness of God. The whole religion of the Hindu is centered in realization. Man is to become divine, realizing the divine, and therefore, idol or temple or church or books, are only the supports, the helps of his spiritual childhood, but on and on he must progress.[149]

In Christianity we not only seek union with God personally and in community, but we also seek to serve the Christ in others, to be a present and active energetic force of love and peace and justice. As we each awaken to the realization of the kingdom of God within, we are empowered to become stronger and more resilient than ever to spread his message of peace, mercy, justice, kindness, love, and compassion to the ends of the earth. The world we live in needs the message of Jesus, and humanity and the earth need our full and complete awakening to his Way of seeing and being— serving, healing, loving—in the world. As the prophet Micah told us, "And what does the Lord require of you but to do justice, and to love kindness, and to walk humbly with your God?" (Micah 6:8).

## My Path to Walk

In responding to the call of Jesus to follow him, I begin each day anew with healing of myself. I receive and give energy through my chakras with a newfound awareness. I heal my body, my memories, and my emotions through every modality available to me—through prayer, worship, yoga *asanas, pranayama*, massage, psychotherapy, spiritual direction, acupuncture, healthy eating, tapping for emotional freedom, and meditation. I call on the Spirit of Jesus to strengthen me, to give me wisdom, to show me the Way so that I may help others. I share what I know so that others can know too and decide for themselves. I give love in the name of Jesus so that others may heal and know that God is love and continues with aliveness and vitality in our time, in our bodies, in our lives.

What is true for me is true for everyone when Christ Consciousness becomes the Way:

The Spirit of God is my breath.

The Spirit of God gives me life.

The Spirit of God pulses through my
body, my veins, my heartbeat.

The Spirit of God quickens my step, enlivens
my hop, my skip, my jump.

The Spirit of God dances with me wildly and freely and
then brings me to quiet where I dissolve into everything.

The Spirit of God moves through my mind and
thoughts when I set my intention toward wisdom,
guidance, and higher consciousness.

The Spirit of God works through my heart when I offer
compassion, when I care for another not because they
care for me but because I see God in their eyes.

The Spirit of God works in my eyes when I see that my
pollution affects your rain, your drinking water.

The Spirit of God works in the eyes of my heart when I see
that my consumerism affects your dignity—for the better
when it gives you work—and when it degrades your dignity,
the Spirit of God helps me see the error of my ways.

The Spirit of God helps me to know when I have
more than enough, and when you are lacking, nudging
me to reach out and make your life better.

The Spirit of God guides me to see that this life is all gift,
pure gift, and is not meant to be lived selfishly, at the
expense or exploitation of others so that I can be more
comfortable—no, the Spirit of God helps me to recognize
when I am needed to help attain the greater good of all.

The Spirit of God opens my soul—my heart, voice,
intuition, and consciousness—to see both beauty and
pain, and to make space for healing and wisdom and
love to emerge from my own actions to others.

The Spirit of God moves me to ask for forgiveness when I have
harmed another or myself, or when I have moved against God.

The Spirit of God brings the integration of all experiences
and forms so that only faith, hope, and love remain,
and above all love, for love is the experience of God's
universal light illuminating all of creation.

It is the Spirit of God that brings me to the Consciousness
of Christ, the Universal Consciousness that is only love.

On my mat, in the cave of my heart, I hear the vibrations of
sympathetic strings that reverberate in my soul. I am a Christian on
the yoga mat. I receive from Christ's table to become and be what I
eat and drink: Christ Consciousness. I move on my mat to awaken
and activate the divine energy within. Breathing in, I am the
sound: *Soooo*. Breathing out, I am the sound: *Haaaammm*. *So Ham*.
*So Ham* in Sanskrit: I am that. I am that I am.
Aum. Om. Amen.

# ~ 12 ~

## YogaMass –
## *Integration Through Ritual and Practice*

Embodied spirituality on the mat, sharing Christ's sacred meal.
—*YogaMass Theme*

### In the Flow

The invitation emails have gone out one last time, and the YogaMass service is but a day away. This is sacred time for me. I like to think of it as going "into the zone," staying intentionally present to the Spirit leading me to what I will say, to how I will lead the flow, to how I will be present in consecrating the bread and wine for the people gathered to become one with the presence of Christ and to become Christ Consciousness. This is a time "set apart" for me to listen closely to God's still, small voice speaking to me in the silence. Dropping into the zone is an intentional move on my part, when I don't allow anything on my calendar and I stay close to my heart. It's actually a very energetic time. I feel my heart: I feel it beating, I feel the energy pulsating throughout my body outward from my heart center, I know my heart is alive and wishing to speak. I sense a palpable presence of God during this preparatory time. I call it flow. The Spirit is flowing around me and through me. In this flow, I glimpse the kingdom of God. This is it. This is the life lived in God, the life of allowing God to be first, to use me, to speak through me. This is a life of prayer. This is my yoga.

I began to understand this when my yoga teacher Amba Stapleton sat with me in the early morning sunlight on the porch swing under the jungle tree canopy of Costa Rica. We could hear the howler monkeys saying good morning and the wild birds singing songs of morning joy. We talked about preparing to teach a yoga class, beyond the sequence of flow or the music selection. We talked about preparing the mind and the heart to enter into the space, lead the class, and lead the meditation. The teacher's experience can be a spiritual practice: a selfless outpouring of her words, energy, and heart for the benefit of others. Because the teacher leads flow and the guided meditation for the class, she does not have the same experience of the flow and the deep meditation herself as the participants do. Consequently, the spiritual nurturing of the teacher must be intentional, beyond the class, to ensure her own quiet time to reflect, renew and restore.

Amba explained to me that teaching a yoga class is like preparing a sermon. Sermon writing, she said to me, is my yoga. I hadn't thought of it that way before. If Yoga means "unity" or "oneness" with the universal consciousness, and practically speaking is a means of balancing and harmonizing the body, mind and emotions, then yes, the practice of sermon writing is yoga. When I write sermons, I pray for the Spirit to flow through me and through my words so I can share what God needs me to convey. Yes, it is my heart integrating with the Spirit "flow," and yes, my own human experience and emotions come through in my sermons, so it is true that my sermons become a co-creation of my heart and God's words, given out to the world. And my husband, Gary, as he prepares our Saturday night meal on "sermon night" is also co-creating with God a healthy meal to nourish and sustain us for our Sunday morning worship experience. So yes, if my sermon writing time is listening to God and co-creating with God, then that time and effort is also my yoga—my unity, my oneness with God. And if my life is given in service to God, then my life is my yoga. This realization was a game-changer for me.

Preparing for YogaMass brings me directly into the flow of God's creative energy. As the final preparation is done, I stand in the space (or sometimes feel the need to sit silently), in awe of what God is doing, how God is using me to express with heart, soul, and body my love for Christ. Barbara Brown Taylor, the beautiful author and Episcopal priest, reminded me and the other students in her sermon at the Seminary of the Southwest how "it is a blessing to be a blessing." My partner in YogaMass, The Rev. Dr. John K. Graham, says, "To not offer the embodied approach to spirituality, we are missing a great opportunity to bless many."

During most Eucharist services as a priest, I wear a long, flowing, white alb or robe wrapped with a rope around my waist and a stole. For YogaMass, I wear white, but not the traditional priestly vestments. I wear white yoga pants and a white yoga top, covered with a flowy, white blouse that allows me to move. I feel free and my spirit is happy. I feel comfortable in my skin, in my body, using my voice. The movement and breathing allow me to get deeply grounded in my own being, in my Self and my body, as a vehicle for God to speak through me. Leading YogaMass makes me feel more alive than ever and that's how I know it's what God is leading me to do. When I describe YogaMass, my face lights up, and as one woman told me, even my cheeks light up, reflecting color and aliveness!

Perhaps my enthusiasm is contagious. Interestingly, the root word for enthusiasm is the Greek word *enthousiasmos*, which stems from *enthous*, meaning, "possessed by a god" or "inspired." The Greek word *theos* is the word used for God in the New Testament. Enthusiasm, the energetic feeling that comes from the heart, means "inspired by God!" What a fabulous way to view life and to view YogaMass, what God has led me to create for an integral approach to embodied spirituality and worship for the God I love. The realization that enthusiasm comes from God once again validates that we are co-creators with God when we feel enthusiasm for our work and service.

One dear friend helps me to stay calm and grounded when I am nervous about the sequence of poses, reminding me that I don't have to be the perfect yoga instructor: "That's not why we are here. We are here to encounter God." During YogaMass, I prayerfully lead the community in an embodied flow of movement and spiritual awareness for becoming Christ Consciousness. YogaMass brings the community to the transformation of awareness Richard Rohr describes as practice-based spirituality:

> "We must return to practice-based spirituality where the vantage point switches *from looking at God to looking out from God.*"[150]

In the experience called YogaMass, it is God's creative energy flowing through us, changing our hearts, perspectives, and our consciousness. My role is simply to hold the space for spiritual experience and to remind everyone present of the great truth of God's love for us in Jesus Christ, and of the presence of God within, the *Imago Dei*. I also intentionally strive to create the inner space for each person to discover and awaken to their path of the Christ Consciousness within, regardless of where they may be on their spiritual journey at that moment.

## Engaging Our Senses In Worship

As the late, great English poet William Blake said in *Marriage of Heaven and Hell*, "The five senses are the chief inlets of the soul." YogaMass is a sensual experience, awakening the senses to engage with soul movement. The Reverend Dr. John K. Graham loves the way YogaMass offers an integral approach to worship using the senses. He says, "We engage all our senses in the Eucharist. The whole person is body, soul, and spirit while the beautiful Eucharist stimulates and touches our heart and our soul. By integrating yoga, we also integrate the body, creating a holistic approach to the mass." The sensuousness of YogaMass is an expression of Jung's *Eros*, or feminine archetypal energy, and it offers a way to connect with the soul and higher consciousness through increasing the inclusive, receptive, open, and adaptive energies of the feminine.

The YogaMass ambience is permeated by the sweet smell of incense from India. A thin white veil with embroidered edging lightly drapes the altar, and two priest stoles gently fall over the table ends. In front of the altar, a candlelit icon of Jesus the Pantocrator (which means "Ruler of All" in Greek) faces the people. Standing near the written image of Christ's face is a wooden cross, hollowed out by natural forces, reminding us of the beauty of imperfection, the gift of grace. The gentle, humming sound of the sitar played by Stuart Nelson fills the space, softly, gently, drawing us in as people gather to place their mats and settle in. Some quietly meditate; others stretch and move at their own rhythm, others greet their friends.

Creating the sacred space for the gathering is important. YogaMass offers, like a yoga studio, open space for mats and flexibility for rearranging the room as needed. The various items that create the altar and the sacred space are treasures gathered from my spiritual pilgrimages and sacred places. The spirituality of YogaMass brings in the five senses of sight, touch, taste, smell, and sound, embodying the creative products of many cultures and traditions.

The service begins with the sounds of the Tibetan bowl ringing out to announce without words that this is sacred space, sacred time, and sacred presence. The soft, rhythmic beat of the djembe drum played by Cyrus Wirls brings a pulse of energy and vibration into the space. Cyrus Wirls and Stuart Nelson, our sitar player, both part of the Institute for Spirituality and Health leadership team, fully embrace the embodied nature of the YogaMass worship experience.

Stuart Nelson describes the significance of the sitar in the creative process of YogaMass as it unfolds during the service:

> The soft, gentle, hum of the drone string, and the bright, sharp, twang of the melody string combine to create a sound unlike any other. And those are just two of 21 strings! Five others get played from time to time, punctuating the raga with dramatic effect, and the player never touches the remaining 14. Instead, they rely on the harmonic resonance of the struck strings to vibrate and create "undertones," further contributing to the distinct sound. Therefore, the mechanics of sitar music are not slave to the hand of the player. They are infused with a creative vibratory connection between the strings themselves.

The vibration of the sympathetic strings flows out to us, and we feel the creative energy rising and flowing among us and within us. Nelson describes this movement of energy from the sounds of the sitar as "literally creating a reverberation outward into the world, echoing into and through the mystery of creation." In YogaMass, the mystery is palpable. We experience the reverberations of creative expression of Spirit flowing in a powerful way.

During the *asana* flow, the gentle sitar music and the rhythmic sound of the djembe drumming help to bring us in touch with our bodies and our feelings as we flow and move and express ourselves. The music communicates the worship of the musicians; Stuart Nelson describes how he deeply resonates with Ravi Shankar, the classical Indian musician and most famous sitar player in the modern era, who said, "The music that I have learned and want to give is like worshipping God. It's absolutely like a prayer." For Nelson, his musical worship flows out from him, with the sound of the sitar lulling him and all of us into a more awakened spiritual state. Nelson on sitar brings into the experience the lineage of yoga's Indian heritage:

> "The sitar is the perfect instrument to feature in YogaMass. It has an allure to it that matured through the centuries alongside yoga itself. Just as the *asanas* featured in the service prepare us to receive the Word, so does the sitar. The sound penetrates the soul and turns the heart toward God."

With the sitar humming, and the djembe rhythms speeding up and slowing down, we flow in synchronization of the sounds with movement and breath. Cyrus Wirls on djembe feels the flow and adds rhythmic beats to awaken the senses, increase energy, and bring us back into a relaxed state with total awareness of what is happening energetically and spiritually within.

During Holy Communion when we receive from the Lord's Table, Taize-style music led by singer and songwriter Diane Davis Andrew gently fills the room with angelic voices, soft guitar, sweet flute melodies, and smooth, silky violin embraces. The Spirit of God speaks through the musicians, singers, and the human hearts gathered, creating a spiritual connection between souls.

We use an Icon of Christ Pantocrator in YogaMass that I brought home with me from a monastery in Meteora, Greece that is perched in the majestic, vertical rock formations and seemingly suspended in the air at a 1,000-foot elevation. The Greek Orthodox monks write the icons as prayer, as work. When I first laid eyes on this depiction of Christ surrounded by archangels around his head, the beauty of the presence of Christ struck me, and I felt his presence as if his eyes reached across the distance to where he could actually "see" me.

There are interpretations of the meaning of this icon. Most traditional icons depict both sides of Jesus' face differently. The icon that spoke to me doesn't reflect a more stern side of him as do most Pantocrator icons; instead, this icon shows a caring, compassionate Christ who can see inside my soul. One interpretation that I appreciate is that the two-dimensional side to Christ's face presents Christ of eternity outside of time and space—his divine nature, while the three-dimensional side presents Christ incarnated into the time and space of creation, his human nature. Both his divine nature and his human nature are joined perfectly in one person at the Incarnation. In YogaMass, we reflect on our own natures, and the divine spark of God within each of us, and as our eyes rest on the Icon of Christ Pantocrator we see the Christ whom we love, gently and compassionately looking back at us, inviting us into the same wholeness of natures.

The delicate white altar linen comes from one of my travels to Israel and into the state of Palestine. High atop the Wadi Qelt that overlooks the road to Jericho live a community of Palestinian Bedouins, selling their handmade wares to tourists. It was here, high up on this mountain, that I celebrated my first Eucharist in Israel. As we were heading down the pathway, the Palestinian men offered to sell us scarves, and silver, turquoise, and coral jewelry. When I spotted the delicate scarf handmade by a Bedouin who lives directly on the land where Jesus walked, I knew this would become a special altar cloth for me, connecting me to the people who humbly live off the land in Palestine, in a manner we in the United States would call impoverished living. My heart saw in the eyes of these men and young boys that they wanted us to not only buy from them but to "see" them, and my response was to want the world to know and remember them, and to see with spiritual eyes that they too, these Muslim men and children, are God's people.

The hollowed out cross is a special cross, carved by a talented woodworker, artist, and member of the Episcopal Diocese of

Texas, Margaret Bailey. Margaret finds interesting pieces of Texas wood and carves crosses out of them. Her crosses are beautiful, and even more importantly, they *feel* good to touch. Margaret didn't create the hollow space in this cross. A living artist created it: the tree. God the Creator spoke through that tree, and the imperfection is beautiful.

When we smell, we engage more deeply into the experience. Burning incense heightens the spirituality of making an offering. "Let my prayer be counted as incense before you, and the lifting up of my hands as the evening sacrifice!" (Psalm 141:2). Priests offer incense around the offerings on the altar. Before YogaMass participants arrive, I say a silent prayer and light the incense, carrying the burning incense I brought from India around the space, filling the room with the scented smoke, and offering prayers for the people who will be arriving. This ritual both clears the energy in the room and prepares it for sacred worship.

The incense bowl is a beautiful hand-made pottery bowl made by the monks of the Society of St. John the Evangelist in Cambridge, Massachusetts, an Episcopal monastic community on the bank of Charles River adjacent to Harvard University. While on retreat there, the monks remained in silence, except for the beautiful chanting offered during worship. Bringing their spirituality into the YogaMass sacred space deepens the experience for me, encouraging me to hold sacred space for those worshiping.

The Eucharistic meal provides a way for us to engage taste and smell, as we taste the bread and drink the wine. The bread and the wine have aromas that invite you to participate and enjoy. Jesus knew we needed to eat, and it is very appropriate that he asked us to remember him when we eat together. It's one way to get us to come together, knowing we would always enjoy a meal! And it's a great way to encourage his friends to remember him often and to stay in community rather than eat alone.

Jesus wanted us to have his heart and his mind, and so we gather with all of our senses, ready and open to become like him, in our own unique way, so that we can be transformed into the heart and mind of Christ himself. Through engagement of our complete selves—bodies, minds, hearts, souls, and spirits—and the recognition that the sacrament of Holy Communion reveals to us the deep truth and reality that Christ is present, YogaMass offers a sensory and fully participative experience of Christ's divine light and consciousness within. Everyone is welcome. We invite people to *come and see, move and breathe, taste and drink, become and be.*

## YogaMass: An Embodied Worship Experience

The Reverend Dr. John K. Graham describes the YogaMass experience as "a heartfelt religious experience that touches our emotions deeply, and our emotions are embedded in our bodies." We experience God somatically through the senses. As the service opens and the sitar music with gentle drumming begins to softly play, we begin to move together in a coordinated flow designed to raise the energy in our bodies and to increase the sensations and awareness of being alive. We feel the touch of our hands on our own bodies as we slide a hand down the leg in *Viparita Virabhadrasana* (Reverse Warrior Pose), or as we clasp our hands together behind our backs and forward fold in Standing Yoga Mudra. I design the flow to ground us in our bodies and increase the energy flow along the spine to open the chakras, helping us to remember to pay attention to our breath and various aspects of our bodies. We open our hip joints to aid in releasing stuck energy, we lengthen our abdomen to align our will with God's will, we open our hearts to love, and we open our throats to speak our truths. We open our third eye to wisdom spoken and felt. We open our crown chakra to receive divine energy and Spirit into our bodies and our hearts. We take the time to touch, feel, experience. We experience the sense of getting in touch with our own subtle energy system. We remember that our bodies are temples for the Spirit within us. We work to release what needs to be released so that love and energy and Spirit within us can flow freely.

The kinesthetic types who feel things to learn experience a deeper worship when their bodies are engaged with *asanas* and *pranayama*. The audio types who need to hear words and music engage on the heart level by listening to the sounds of the soft sitar, the rhythmic djembe drumming, Spirit-filled chanting, instructional guidance for breath and movement, the words of Holy Scripture and Holy Communion, guided meditation, and *savasana*. The visual types see the elements of ritual—the mat, musicians and singers, the Bible, the incense smoke gently rising, the plate of bread, the cup of wine—and engage with a sense of understanding and inclusion in a community of faith.

After movement, heart openers, and *pranayama*, we stand tall and still in mountain pose to hear the gospel, and we sit to hear a short message that reflects on the teaching. We move again in a guided flow in response to the teaching. What is God saying to us? How can we incorporate the message beyond our thinking minds into our hearts and bodies? I lead us in reflective questions such as, "What is God calling you to let go of?" and "How is God calling you to align your will with the holy?" Feeling the presence of the holy in your breath, in your body, creates an experience of awareness of the divine. We prepare ourselves to receive from the Lord's Table through opening our bodies and paying attention to where we are now, and where we want to be physically, emotionally, intellectually, energetically, and spiritually.

Engaging in worship as a sensual experience is an embodied approach to spirituality through the body, its energies, and the soul. The worship experience would not be complete without verbal expression, so that in community we come into the same mind, a oneness of Christ Consciousness. This integral approach to worship of engaging the body in sensual experience and using words for communication and understanding is an expression of Jung's *Eros* and *Logos*—the experience itself as *Eros*, and bringing it into consciousness through words as *Logos*. It is also harmonious with the yogic understanding of awareness of body and mind consciousness.

Full participation in the worship and devotion for God in experience and consciousness brings us into a greater wholeness. We seek something greater than ourselves—we seek wholeness, we seek healing, we seek God who can do for us what we can't do for ourselves. We come together to experience a deep sense of belonging, with an understanding and a commitment: *this is my story and these are my people.* I belong. The ritual of encountering God together in a community meets the *Eros* archetypal need for connection and being included in something greater than ourselves, and helps us to see that God's vision is greater than what any of us can do alone. We need each other, not only in our work and service for others, but also for our own healing and journey to wholeness. We come, we see, we hear, we taste, we are nourished, and then we go back out into the world restored, renewed, rejuvenated to do the work God has given us to do.

One aspect that makes YogaMass unique is the relationship of all the people gathered together in community, each individual fully participating, or as much as they choose or are able to do so. The Reverend Dr. John K. Graham from the Institute for Spirituality and Health at the Texas Medical Center and I work together in a spiritual flow, co-officiating the worship experience. The musicians and vocalists from the Institute for Spirituality and Health, Grace Episcopal Church, and friends, join with us in that flow as we invite the Holy Spirit into our midst. All the people who are leading the worship experience come with open hearts and expectations that God will show up. There is no sense of competition, and the gathered community is open to each other and to God's Holy Spirit. Something deeply moving happens as a result of our openness: there is a palpable sense of God's presence and movement through us, in and among us.

Everyone in the worship community adds to the experience. We open and we receive what God has to offer us. We know energetically when the Spirit is moving, because we feel the hairs on our arms stand up, and tears begin to flow. The movement, the music, the sensory stimulations draw us in deeper. The creative nature of our collective experience flows from us and between us, not planned but free, with no expectations, simply response to Spirit.

When we say the Eucharistic prayer, it is a collective prayer. Different people each time stand and speak the words from the Eucharistic prayer. When the priests and the people gathered all participate in offering the Eucharistic prayer, everyone is invited more deeply into the experience of Jesus' life and path. It is our collective voice, us, not one or two mediating for the whole. In essence, we become "The Body" of Christ: one body, one voice, one heart. Unity in diversity—celebrating the divine, celebrating Jesus' humanity. The YogaMass theme comes alive: "Embodied spirituality on the mat, sharing Christ's sacred meal." We participate in the divine liturgy of the Eucharist on a personal level, integrating the words of Jesus into our own life, offering ourselves up to a greater reality: "This is my body, given for you." My heart vibrates with joy as the words of Jesus become our own.

The integral approach of bringing yoga into the Holy Communion worship experience invites our entire Self into the experience as an offering to God. The mind gets quiet when focusing on the breath, the movements, and the stillness in between, better able to focus on the words of Holy Scripture and words of Institution as the bread and wine are consecrated to become the holy presence of Christ. The participants' hearts physically, energetically, and spiritually open to God, and are enveloped in the presence of the holy. We taste the mystical body and blood of Christ within us and among us, an experience of union with Christ in sacred community.

Participants are inspired to discover a deeper faith in Christ, which brings a deep acceptance and joy that I have not been able to find another way. The mystical Christ among us and within me shows me the way. The compassion of Christ heals us and helps us to encounter God in the other. People share after the service that they feel peaceful. When peace is flowing, it's a sure sign that the Holy Spirit is present and moving among us.

YogaMass gives space for a renewed spirituality based on Christ's own realization of the presence of the divine within. Jesus leads us to this realization for ourselves. We integrate the presence of God into our bodies and our soul consciousness in a holistic way, just as Jesus did. The presence of Christ is among us, and within us, and we are empowered to live in a new way, with a renewed sense of God's Spirit within us, ready to share the love of Christ with those around us. This experience often fulfills what Jesus desired for those who love him:

> "As the Father has loved me, so I have loved you; abide in my love. If you keep my commandments, you will abide in my love, just as I have kept my Father's commandments and abide in his love. I have said these things to you so that my joy may be in you, and that your joy may be complete" (John 15:9-11).

We come ready to experience life: to move, to breathe, to feel, to become, to be. One participant, Anyang Anyang, shared why YogaMass has been important in his faith journey: "I was able to re-discover so many truths in Christianity that I had taken for granted, and YogaMass provided a perfect opportunity for me to carry that spirit of embodiment. I have re-discovered Christianity and the love of Christ in a very visceral sense."

As we come to know ourselves more fully, we gain the capacity to go deeper and deeper in the love that Jesus imparts to us and to become that same love. Abiding in his love begins with the realization that we are simultaneously physical, psychological, social, and spiritual beings, and that our very createdness integrates these components for our human experience to fully manifest. In our fullness, we awaken and rise to a greater and higher consciousness, and ultimately, by grace, we awaken to Christ Consciousness. Living in higher consciousness takes us beyond ourselves, reaching out to bring those around us to an awakened state of being. Our lives then become a living prayer to help others see that the kingdom of heaven is, in fact, within us.

At the end of YogaMass, with hands in prayer over my heart, I bow to the beautiful people around me and say,

*"Peace be with you. The divine light in me bows to the divine light in you. Namaste."*

And we all bow to each other in deep gratitude.

This is embodied love.

# Appendix

# YogaMass Liturgy

For many Christians, the experience of God—and most especially in worship—comes from the mind, or intellect. From the Enlightenment period forward, this has been the path of the Western Church and Western culture. We use our minds, valuing mostly our ability to understand, think, and know everything from a scientific and knowledge perspective, including God. Mystics know there is more. The longest journey is from the head to the heart, with the journey's goal being to experience God with one's whole heart. From a heart perspective, the experience of God is a deep, inner knowing with a palpable feeling of the presence of love and light.

Entering into the worship experience with the body through YogaMass prepares one for a worship experience beyond the head and into the heart, the organ of cosmic consciousness. It includes all of the physical body—the energetic body, and the yogic subtle bodies—and the mind, soul, and spirit, all engaging together in expression of the whole person. When we engage the body into the worship experience through the use of *asanas, pranayama*, and meditation, we engage ourselves more fully in the experience, and we more fully integrate our devotion to God as a holistic expression of all that we are—body, mind (thoughts and feelings), soul (intuition and consciousness), and spirit, propelling us upward toward Christ Consciousness.

The YogaMass liturgy is an approved Holy Eucharist, Rite III liturgy in the Episcopal Diocese of Texas, authorized by The Right Reverend C. Andrew Doyle, IX Bishop of Texas. I am grateful to all those who helped shape it into what it has become, and to all those who will guide this movement going forward. I am especially grateful to The Reverend Dr. John K. Graham for his inclusive vision, his encouragement to write this book, and for his team at the Institute for Spirituality and Health at the Texas Medical Center. I am grateful to The Reverend Dr. Stephen Kinney of The Front Porch in Austin, Texas, an Episcopal worshipping community, for his contribution in the Eucharistic prayer of the YogaMass liturgy. I am also grateful to all of the YogaMass participants for your willingness to open to God in this beautiful way. Thanks be to God from whom all blessings flow.

The YogaMass liturgy below is offered for your reference. You may use it for creating your own YogaMass worship experience upon obtaining copyright permission. I invite you to experience embodied spirituality in the way of YogaMass. Please visit our website, **yogamass.com**, for more information and for upcoming events.I look forward to meeting you on your yoga mat near the altar of our hearts.

Thank you for your open mind and open heart.

The divine light in me bows to the divine light in you. Namaste.

# YogaMass

GATHERING

## WELCOME AND INVITATION
*deep listening and dialogue with God*

## YOGA
*guided gentle flow movement or flow as inner-directed*

## GOSPEL OR EPISTLE READING
*(standing)*

## RESPONSE TO THE WORD
*guided reflection through meditation in motion and breath*

## THE EUCHARISTIC CELEBRATION
*honoring the deep mysteries of God (seated)*

What we are looking for is already here.
**Blessed are the hungry ones, for our inner longings will be satisfied.**

Lift up your hearts.
**We lift up our hearts to you, O God, and give thanks, and we bow our heads to You, and to our own hearts, honoring your divine light shining upon us and within us, and upon all of creation.**

Jesus came to bring Light into the world, to teach people the truth of God's love for them and for all people, and the truth of living in God's presence.

He walked in Light, sharing his power and his Spirit by healing, teaching, sharing meals, and feeding the crowds with the food that brings true life.

He had compassion for the lonely, the sick, the brokenhearted, the poor, the naked, the imprisoned, and he asked his friends to care for them as much as they cared for themselves.

Around his table, every life mattered...whether one was religious or pagan, man or woman, young or old, sinner or saint.

Around the table, people met at the level of their most basic need—not just for food, but also for each other.

And so we gather at this table.

We remember the stories of bread broken and shared, of Jesus feeding the crowds, of unlikely guests revealing the face of God.

It was on a night of both celebration and betrayal that he took the bread leftover on the table, blessed it, broke it, and gave it as his body given for them.
This is my body.

Then he took the cup also leftover on the table, and shared it with them as his blood, to be the life given for the life of the world.
This is my blood.

He stood in his truth, and he offered himself as a witness to the power of love, showing us the way to true life.

Breathe upon us, Spirit of life, and upon this bread and this wine, that we may burn with your Spirit's power. Unite us to you and your Son Jesus, with His Spirit, that we all may be one.

Let us join our voices and pray together.

*Giver of Life, draw us together and bring us to wholeness, so that your light shines in us and through us, in our creations and out into the world, in the Spirit of Christ. AMEN.*

## SHARING THE PEACE
Recognizing our oneness, let us greet one another in love.
*stand and share the peace of Christ with each other*

## THE BREAKING OF THE BREAD
Christ speaks to us: "I AM IN YOU. YOU ARE IN ME."
"Live in me and I will live in you." (John 15:4)

## SHARING THE GIFTS OF GOD
*the priest continues...*
The gifts of God for the people of God. Take them and become them.
**When you give birth to that which is within yourself, what you bring forth will save you.** (The Gospel of Thomas, Logion 70)

*Communion is shared*
*please come forward to receive the gifts of God, being respectful of sacred space on the mats*

## RESPONSE TO THE GIFTS
*while communion is shared, sit in stillness or flow as inner-directed*

## BREATHING & MEDITATION *(seated)*

## RELAXATION / SAVASANA

## BLESSING & SENDING FORTH OF THE FAITHFUL
The divine Spirit dwells in us.
**Thanks be to God.**
Go now to love and serve the Lord. Go in peace.

*Amen. We go in the name of Christ who dwells in us.*

THANK YOU FOR JOINING US
PEACE, SHANTI, SHALOM, NAMASTE

GRACE EPISCOPAL CHURCH, HOUSTON
THE REVEREND GENA DAVIS

THE INSTITUTE FOR SPIRIUTALITY AND HEALTH
THE REVEREND DR. JOHN K. GRAHAM

The Eucharistic liturgy adapted with permission from The Reverend Dr. Stephen Kinney, The Front Porch, Austin, Texas

# Endnotes

## Introduction

1. Brown, Brené, *Daring Greatly: How the Courage to Be Vulnerable Transforms the Way We Live, Love, Parent, and Lead* (New York: Avery, Penguin Random House, 2012), 92.

2. Consiglio, Cyprian, *Spirit, Soul, Body: Toward an Integral Christian Spirituality* (Copyright 2015 by Order of St. Benedict. Published by Liturgical Press, Collegeville Minnesota), 73. Used with permission.

3. Ibid., 73–74. Used with permission.

4. Webber, Christopher L., *Welcome to the Episcopal Church: An Introduction to Its History, Faith, and Worship* (Harrisburg, Pennsylvania: Morehouse Publishing, 1999), 71.

## Chapter 1: The Birthing of YogaMass – *Creativity and Courage*

5. Tickle, Phyllis, *The Great Emergence: How Christianity is Changing and Why* (Grand Rapids, Michigan: Baker Books, a division of Baker Publishing Group, 2008), 120. Used by permission.

6. Ibid., 25. Used by permission.

7. Ibid., 51. Used by permission.

8. Ibid., 67. Used by permission.

9. Ibid., 96. Used by permission.

10. Ibid., 72. Used by permission.

11. Ibid., 73. Used by permission.

12. Chittister, Joan, O.S.B., *The Rule of Benedict: Insight for the Ages* (New York, New York: The Crossroad Publishing Company, 1992, 2002), 19.

13. Oliver, Mary, *New and Selected Poems: Volume Two* (Boston: Beacon Press, 2005), 4. Reprinted by permission of The Charlotte Sheedy Literary Agency Inc.

## Chapter 2: Engaging Aliveness – *Being Fully Human*

14. Muller, Wayne, *Sabbath: Finding Rest, Renewal, and Delight in our Busy Lives* (New York, NY: Bantam Books, 1999), 21.

15. Chittister, Joan, O.S.B., *The Rule of Benedict: Insights for the Ages* (New York: The Crossroad Publishing Company: 2002), 23–24.

16. Douglas-Klotz, Neil, *Prayers of the Cosmos: Meditations on the Aramaic Words of Jesus*, Brief quote from p. 21, Copyright © 1990 by Neil Douglas-Klotz. Foreword by Matthew Fox. Reprinted by permission of HarperCollins Publishers.

17. Saraswati, Swami Satyananda, *Asana Pranayama Mudra Bandha* (Munger, Bihar, India: Yoga Publications Trust, 1969, 1973, 1996, 2008), 9.

18. Myss, Caroline, PhD., *Anatomy of the Spirit: The Seven Stages of Power and Healing* (New York: Crown Publishers, Inc., 1996), 66–67.

19. Ibid., 67.

20. Douglas-Klotz, Neil, *Prayers of the Cosmos: Meditations on the Aramaic Words of Jesus*, Brief quote from p. 21, Copyright © 1990 by Neil

Douglas-Klotz. Foreword by Matthew Fox. Reprinted by permission of HarperCollins Publishers.

21. Wilber, Ken, *Integral Spirituality: A Startling New Role for Religion in the Modern and Postmodern World* (Boston, Massachusetts: Integral Books, 2006), 16.

22. Rohr, Richard, *The Naked Now: Learning to See as the Mystics See* (New York: The Crossroads Publishing Company, 2009), 29-30.

## Chapter 3: The Inner Landscape – *The Crucial Pilgrimage*

23. Julian of Norwich in *All Will be Well: Julian of Norwich*, compiler Richard Chilson (Notre Dame, Indiana: Ave Maria Press, 1995, 2008), 66.

24. Hastings, Adrian, Editor, *The Oxford Companion to Christian Thought* (Oxford: Oxford University Press, 2000), 541.

25. Oliver, Mary, *New and Selected Poems: Volume Two* (Boston, Massachusetts: Beacon Press, 2005), 86. Reprinted by permission of The Charlotte Sheedy Literary Agency Inc.

26. Judith, Anodea, *Chakra Activation* (Boulder, Colorado: Sounds True, soundstrue.com, 2011).

27. Schulte, Brigid, (2015, May 26), "Harvard Neuroscientist: Meditation not only reduces stress, here's how it changes your brain." *The Washington Post*, 2-3.

28. Seager, Richard Hughes, *The World's Parliament of Religions: The East/West Encounter, Chicago, 1893* (Indiana: Indiana University Press, 1995), p. viii.

29. Trungpa, Chögyam, *Shambhala: The Sacred Path of the Warrior* (Boston, Massachusetts: Shambhala Publications, Inc., 1984), 20-21.

30. Freeman, Laurence, OSB, *Light Within: The Inner Path of Meditation* (New York, New York: The Crossroad Publishing Company, 1986), 19.

31. "Forget Your Life" from THE ILLUMINATED RUMI by Jalal Al-Din Rumi, copyright © 1997 by Coleman Barks and Michael Green. Used by permission of Broadway Books, an imprint of the Crown Publishing Group, a division of Penguin Random House LLC. All rights reserved.

## Chapter 4: Self-Discovery – *Finding the True Self*

32. Keating, Thomas, *The Human Condition: Contemplation and Transformation* (New York, New York: Paulist Press, 1999), 44.

33. Urbanczik, Aleš, Structural Integration—Ida Rolf's Quest for Balance between Gravity and Man (Santa Cruz, California: A Presentation for the Conference "Learning from others—better holistic understanding" in Dresden, Germany, June 3, 2000).

34. *Journal of Analytic Psychology: The I Ching and the psyche-body connection* (April, 2005), 237-250.

35. Bourgeault, Cynthia, *The Wisdom Jesus: Transforming Heart and Mind—a New Perspective on Christ and His Message* (Boston, Massachusetts: Shambhala Publications, Inc., 2008), 21. Reprinted by arrangement with Shambhala Publications, Inc., Boulder, CO. www.shambhala.com.

36. Bourgeault, Cynthia, *The Meaning of Mary Magdalene: Discovering the Woman at the Heart of Christianity* (Boston, Massachusetts: Shambhala Publications, Inc., Boston, Massachusetts, 2010), 34. Reprinted by arrangement with Shambhala Publications, Inc., Boulder, CO. www.shambhala.com.

37. Wink, Walter, *Unmasking the Powers: The Invisible Forces That Determine Human Existence* (Philadelphia: Fortress Press, 1986), 1.

38. King, Karen L., *The Gospel of Mary of Magdala: Jesus and the First Woman Apostle* (Santa Rosa, California: Polebridge Press, 2003), 189.

39. Bauman, Lynn C., Bauman Ward J., and Bourgeault, Cynthia, *The Luminous Gospels: Thomas, Mary Magdalene, and Philip* (Telephone, Texas: Praxis Publishing, 2008), ix–x. Reprinted by permission.

40. Ibid., x–xi. Reprinted by permission.

41. Arnold, Kenneth, *The Circle of the Way: Reading the Gospel of Thomas as a Christzen Text* (Cross Currents, Winter 2002, Vol. 51, No 4).

42. Bourgeault, Cynthia, *The Gospel of Thomas with Cynthia Bourgeault* (e-Courses@SpiritualityandPractice.com: April 8-May 11, 2013).

43. Meyer, Marvin W., (New Translation, with Introduction and Notes), *The Gospel of Thomas: The Hidden Sayings of Jesus,* Interpretation by Harold Bloom (San Francisco: HarperSanFrancisco, 1992), 112.

44. Bourgeault, Cynthia, *The Wisdom Jesus* (Boston, Massachusetts: Shambhala Publications, Inc.: 2008), 24. Reprinted by arrangement with Shambhala Publications, Inc., Boulder, CO. www.shambhala.com.

45. Rohr, Richard, *Immortal Diamond: The Search for Our True Self* (San Francisco, California: Jossey-Bass, 2013), 36-38. Reprinted by permission.

46. Rohr, Richard, *The Naked Now: Learning to See as the Mystics See* (New York: The Crossroads Publishing Company, 2009), 69.

47. Farhi, Donna, *Yoga Mind, Body, and Spirit: A Return to Wholeness* (New York, New York: St. Martin's Press, 2000), 5.

48. Griffiths, Bede, *Return to the Center* (Springfield, Illinois: Templegate, 1976), 137–139. Reprinted by permission.

49. Lipka, Michael, *A closer look at America's rapidly growing religious 'nones'* (Pew Research Center, May 13, 2015).

50. Masci David, and Lipka, Michael, *Americans may be getting less religious, but feelings of spirituality are on the rise* (Pew Research Center, January 21, 2016).

51. Griffiths, Bede, *Return to the Center,* (Springfield, Illinois: Templegate, 1976), 115. Reprinted by permission.

## Chapter 5: Wholeness and Union – *Goals of the Spiritual Life*

52. Bauman, Lynn C., Bauman Ward J., and Bourgeault, Cynthia, *The Luminous Gospels: Thomas, Mary Magdalene, and Philip* (Telephone, Texas: Praxis Publishing, 2008), 66. Reprinted by permission.

53. Yogananda, Paramahansa, *The Second Coming of Christ: The Resurrection of the Christ Within You, Volume I* (Los Angeles, California: Self-Realization Fellowship, 2004), 804.

54. Pert, Candace, *Molecules of Emotion: The Science behind Mind-Body Medicine* (http://candacepert.com).

55. Ibid.

56. Frawley, David, *Yoga & Ayurveda: Self-Healing and Self-Realization* (Twin Lakes, Wisconsin: Lotus Press, 1999), 149.

57. Ibid., 152.

58. Bauman, Lynn C., Bauman Ward J., and Bourgeault, Cynthia, *The Luminous Gospels: Thomas, Mary Magdalene, and Philip* (Telephone, Texas: Praxis Publishing, 2008), 95. Reprinted by permission.

59. Saraswati, Swami Satyananda, *Asana Pranayama Mudra Bandha* (Munger, Bihar, India: Yoga Publications Trust, 1969, 1973, 1996, 2008), 1.

60. Ibid.

61. Ibid., 2–3.

62. Ibid., 3.

63. Spong, John Shelby, *A New Christianity for a New World* (Morristown, New Jersey: Christianity for the Third Millennium), 21–22.

64. Ibid., 35.

65. Borg, Marcus J., *Jesus: Uncovering the Life, Teachings, and Relevance of a Religious Revolutionary* (New York, New York: HarperCollins Publishers, 2006), 222.

## Chapter 6: Making the Ancient New (Again) – *Returning to Soul*

66. Yogananda, Paramahansa, *The Yoga of Jesus* (Los Angeles, California: Self-Realization Fellowship, 2007, 2014), 80. Used by permission.

67. Notovitch, Nicolas, *The Unknown Life of Jesus Christ* (Chicago, Illinois: Indo-American Book Company, 1894), 92.

68. Yogananda, Paramahansa, *The Yoga of Jesus* (Los Angeles, California: Self-Realization Fellowship, 2007, 2014), 81. Used by permission.

69. Bauman, Lynn C., Bauman Ward J., and Bourgeault, Cynthia, *The Luminous Gospels: Thomas, Mary Magdalene, and Philip* (Telephone, Texas: Praxis Publishing, 2008), 59. Reprinted by permission.

70. Satchidananda, Sri Swami, *The Yoga Sutras of Patanjali* (Buckingham, Virginia: The Yoga Sutras of Patanjali, 1978, 2011, 2012, 2015), xii.

71. Iyengar, B.K.S., *Light on Yoga* (New York: Schoken Books, 1966, 1968, 1976, 1977, 1978), 22.

72. Ibid.

73. Chittister, Joan, O.S.B., *The Rule of Benedict: Insights for the Ages* (New York: The Crossroad Publishing Company: 2002), 66.

74. Artress, Lauren, *Walking a Sacred Path: Rediscovering the Labyrinth as a Spiritual Practice* (New York: Riverhead Books, 1995), 135. Used by permission of Riverhead, an imprint of Penguin Publishing Group, a division of Penguin Random House LLC. All rights reserved.

## Chapter 7: Awakening – *Healing and Inner Knowing*

75. McGehee, J. Pittman and Thomas, Damon J., *The Invisible Church: Finding Spirituality Where You Are,* (Westport, Connecticut, London: Praeger, 2009), 59. Used by permission.

76. Swami Satyananda Saraswati, *Prana: The Universal Life Force* (Zinal, Switzerland: yogamag.net, September 1981).

77. Judith, Anodea, *Eastern Body, Western Mind: Psychology and the Chakra System as a Path to the Self* (Berkeley, CA: Celestial Arts, 1996, 2004), 4–5. Used by permission of Celestial Arts, an imprint of the Crown Publishing Group, a division of Penguin Random House LLC. All rights reserved.

78. Ibid., 12-13. Used by permission.

79. Ibid., 5. Used by permission.

80. Wilber, Ken, *Integral Spirituality: A Startling New Role for Religion in the Modern and Postmodern World* (Boston, Massachusetts: Integral Books, 2006), 13.

81. Judith, Anodea, *Eastern Body, Western Mind: Psychology and the Chakra System as a Path to the Self* (Berkeley, CA: Celestial Arts, 1996, 2004), 5. Used by permission of Celestial Arts, an imprint of the Crown

Publishing Group, a division of Penguin Random House LLC. All rights reserved.

82. Jung, C. G., *Memories, Dreams, Reflections* (New York: Random House, Inc., 1961, 1962, 1963).

83. Marion, Jim, *Putting on the Mind of Christ: The Inner Work of Christian Spirituality* (Charlottesville, Virginia: Hampton Roads Publishing Company, Inc., 2000), 192.

84. Yogananda, Paramahansa, *The Yoga of Jesus* (Los Angeles, California: Self-Realization Fellowship, 2007, 2014), 30. Used by permission.

85. Hanh, Thich Nhat, *Old Path White Clouds: Walking in the Footsteps of the Buddha* (Berkeley, California: Parallax Press, 1991), p. 213.

86. Griffiths, Bede, *The Marriage of East and West* (Springfield, Illinois: Templegate Publishers, 1982), 167. Reprinted by permission.

## Chapter 8: Embodied Spirituality – *Incarnation*

87. Rohr, Richard, *Things Hidden: Scripture as Spirituality* (Cincinnati, Ohio: St. Anthony Messenger Press, 2008), 17.

88. Bourgeault, Cynthia, *The Meaning of Mary Magdalene: Discovering the Woman at the Heart of Christianity* (Boston, Massachusetts: Shambhala Publications, Inc., Boston, Massachusetts, 2010), 63-64. Reprinted by arrangement with Shambhala Publications, Inc., Boulder, CO. www.shambhala.com.

89. Cross, F.L. and Livingstone, E. A., *The Oxford Dictionary of the Christian Church, Third Edition Revised* (Oxford: Oxford University Press, 2005), 830.

90. Ibid., 998.

91. Ibid.

92. Fox, Matthew, *The Coming of the Cosmic Christ: The Healing of Mother Earth and the Birth of a Global Renaissance*, Brief quote from pp. 94-5 from THE COMING OF THE COSMIC CHRIST by MATTHEW FOX. Copyright © 1988 Matthew Fox. Reprinted by permission of HarperCollins Publishers.

93. Cross, F.L. and Livingstone, E. A., *The Oxford Dictionary of the Christian Church, Third Edition Revised* (Oxford: Oxford University Press, 2005), 335.

94. Yogananda, Paramahansa, *The Second Coming of Christ, Volume II* (Los Angeles, California: Self-Realization Fellowship, 2004), 912. Used by permission.

95. Bourgeault, Cynthia, *The Meaning of Mary Magdalene: Discovering the Woman at the Heart of Christianity* (Boston, Massachusetts: Shambhala Publications, Inc., Boston, Massachusetts, 2010), 177–178. Reprinted by arrangement with Shambhala Publications, Inc., Boulder, CO. www. shambhala.com.

96. Ibid., 217.

97. Ibid., 61.

98. Nhat Hanh, Thich, *Living Buddha, Living Christ* (New York: Riverhead Books, 1995), 123.

99. Bauman, Lynn C., Bauman Ward J., and Bourgeault, Cynthia, *The Luminous Gospels: Thomas, Mary Magdalene, and Philip* (Telephone, Texas: Praxis Publishing, 2008), 105. Reprinted by permission.

100. Merton, Thomas, *Conjectures of an Innocent Bystander* (Garden City, New York: Doubleday, 1968, 1969), 158.

101. Consiglio, Cyprian, *Spirit, Soul, Body: Toward an Integral Christian Spirituality* (Copyright 2015 by Order of St. Benedict. Published by Liturgical Press, Collegeville Minnesota), 73. Used with permission.

102. Richard Rohr, *Immortal Diamond: The Search for Our True Self* (Jossey-Bass: 2013), 38-39. Reprinted by permission.

## Chapter 9: Living in the Flow - *Surrender*

103. Gates, Rolf, and Kenison, Katrina, *Meditations from the Mat: Daily Reflections on the Path of Yoga* (New York: Anchor Books, 2002), 317.

104. Adele, Deborah, *The Yamas and the Niyamas: Exploring Yoga's Ethical Practice* (Duluth, Minnesota: On-Word Bound Books LLC), 93–94.

105. Chittister, Joan, O.S.B., *The Rule of Benedict: Insights for the Ages* (New York, New York: The Crossroad Publishing Company, 1992), 172-173.

106. Hanh, Thich Nhat, *How to Walk* (Berkeley, California: Parallax Press, 2015), 31.

107. Gates, Rolf, and Kenison, Katrina, *Meditations from the Mat: Daily Reflections on the Path of Yoga* (New York: Anchor Books, 2002), 241.

108. Artress, Lauren, *Walking a Sacred Path: Rediscovering the Labyrinth as a Spiritual Practice* (New York: Riverhead Books, 1995), xv. Used by permission of Riverhead, an imprint of Penguin Publishing Group, a division of Penguin Random House LLC. All rights reserved.

109. Ibid., 86. Used by permission of Riverhead, an imprint of Penguin Publishing Group, a division of Penguin Random House LLC. All rights reserved.

110. Ibid.

111. Gates, Rolf, and Kenison, Katrina, *Meditations from the Mat: Daily Reflections on the Path of Yoga* (New York: Anchor Books, 2002), 86.

112. Artress, Lauren, *Walking a Sacred Path: Rediscovering the Labyrinth as a Spiritual Practice* (New York: Riverhead Books, 1995, 2006), 124-125. Used by permission of Riverhead, an imprint of Penguin Publishing Group, a division of Penguin Random House LLC. All rights reserved.

113. Chopra, Deepak, *Reinventing the Body, Resurrecting the Soul* (New York: Three Rivers Press, an imprint of the Crown Publishing Group, a division of Random House, Inc., 2009), 12.

114. Ibid., 184.

115. Bourgeault, Cynthia, *The Wisdom Way of Knowing: Reclaiming an Ancient Tradition to Awaken the Heart* (San Francisco, CA: Jossey-Bass, 2003), 72.

## Chapter 10: Sacred Ritual – *The Eucharist*

116. McGehee, J. Pittman and Thomas, Damon J., *The Invisible Church: Finding Spirituality Where You Are,* (Westport, Connecticut, London: Praeger, 2009), 59. Used by permission.

117. Rappaport, Roy A., *Ecology, Meaning and Religion* (Richmond, Calif.: North Atlantic Books, 1979), 174. [Emphasis in the original].

118. Pitre, Brant, *Jesus and the Jewish Roots of the Eucharist: Unlocking the Secrets of the Last Supper* (New York: Doubleday Religion, 2011), 71.

119. Chopra, Deepak, *Reinventing the Body, Resurrecting the Soul* (New York: Three Rivers Press, 2009), 8.

120. Griffiths, Bede, *Return to the Center* (Springfield, Illinois: Templegate, 1976), 114. Reprinted by permission.

121. Ibid., 115. Reprinted by permission.

122. Ibid. Reprinted by permission.

123. Keating, Thomas, *The Better Part* (New York: The Continuum International Publishing Group, Inc., 2000), 55-56.

124. Rohr, Richard, OFM, *Eucharist as Touchstone* (Albuquerque, New Mexico: Center for Action and Contemplation, 2000), CD.

## Chapter 11: Awakening into Christ Consciousness – *The Life Teaching of Jesus*

125. Yogananda, Paramahansa, *The Second Coming of Christ: The Resurrection of Christ Within you, Volume I* (Los Angeles, California: Self-Realization Fellowship, 2004), 279–280. Used by permission.

126. Ibid., xxi. Used by permission.

127. Smith, Paul, https://integrallife.com/integral-post/what-christ-consciousness

128. www.desiringgod.org/blog/posts/god-consciousness-is-christ-consciousness

129. www.dlshq.org/religions/christconscious

130. Fox, Matthew, *The Coming of the Cosmic Christ: The Healing of Mother Earth and the Birth of a Global Renaissance,* Brief quote from p. 65 from THE COMING OF THE COSMIC CHRIST by MATTHEW FOX. Copyright © 1988 Matthew Fox. Reprinted by permission of HarperCollins Publishers.

131. Marion, Jim, *Putting on the Mind of Christ: The Inner Work of Christian Spirituality* (Charlottesville, Virginia: Hampton Roads Publishing Company, Inc., 2000), 183.

132. Yogananda, Paramahansa, *The Yoga of Jesus: Understanding the Hidden Teachings of the Gospels* (Los Angeles, California: Self-Realization Fellowship, 2007, 2014), 5. Used by permission.

133. Ibid. Used by permission.

134. Yogananda, Paramahansa, *The Second Coming of Christ, Volume I* (Los Angeles, California: Self-Realization Fellowship, 2004), xxi. Used by permission.

135. Griffiths, Bede, *The Marriage of East and West* (Springfield, Illinois: Templegate Publishers, 1982), 189. Reprinted by permission.

136. Yogananda, Paramahansa, *The Second Coming of Christ: The Resurrection of the Christ Within You, Volume I* (Los Angeles, California: Self-Realization Fellowship, 2004), xxiii. Used by permission.

137. Yogananda, Paramahansa, *The Second Coming of Christ: The Resurrection of the Christ Within You, Volume II* (Los Angeles, California: Self-Realization Fellowship, 2004), 1395. Used by permission.

138. Judith, Anodea, *Eastern Body, Western Mind: Psychology and the Chakra System as a Path to the Self* (Berkeley, CA: Celestial Arts, 1996, 2004), 12-13. Used by permission of Celestial Arts, an imprint of the Crown Publishing Group, a division of Penguin Random House LLC. All rights reserved.

139. Farhat, Amal, *Trumpet Universe and Ascension to the Light and 2012* (eBook: RoseDog Books, 2010), 30.

140. This is How a Human Being Can Change" from THE ILLUMINATED RUMI by Jalal Al-Din Rumi, copyright © 1997 by Coleman Barks and Michael Green. Used by permission of Broadway Books, an imprint of the Crown Publishing Group, a division of Penguin Random House LLC. All rights reserved.

141. Griffiths, Bede, *The Marriage of East and West* (Springfield, Illinois: Templegate Publishers, 1982), 167. Reprinted by permission.

142. Wilber, Ken, *Integral Spirituality: A Startling New Role for Religion in the Modern and Postmodern World* (Boston, Massachusetts: Integral Books, 2006), 14.

143. Griffiths, Bede, *The Marriage of East and West* (Springfield, Illinois: Templegate Publishers, 1982), 198–199. Reprinted by permission.

144. Nhat Hanh, Thich, *Living Buddha, Living Christ* (New York, New York: Riverhead Books, 1995), 58.

145. Teilhard de Chardin, Pierre, *The Future of Man* (Image Books: 1964), 186.

146. Rohr, Richard, *Christ, Cosmology, & Consciousness: A Reframing of How We See* (CAC: 2010), MP3 download.

147. Seager, Richard Hughes, *The World's Parliament of Religions: The East/West Encounter, Chicago, 1893* (Bloomington, Indiana: Indiana University Press, 1995), 110.

148. Ibid., 111–112.

149. Ibid., 112.

## Chapter 12: YogaMass – *Integration through Ritual and Practice*

150. Rohr, Richard, *Immortal Diamond: The Search for Our True Self* (San Francisco, California: Jossey-Bass: 2013), xxiv. Reprinted by permission.